FROM PAIN TO WELLNESS:
Overcoming Autoimmune Diseases, An Undisclosed Epidemic

Ionelia Silvia Prajescu

To say thanks for buying this book I would like to send you for free the full list of AIP friendly ingredients and AIP recipes that I publish weekly. If you are interested, please send me a message at

info@aipwellnessjourney.com

You can find my recipes and health tips at

https://aipwellnessjourney.com

or follow my YouTube channel:

AIP Wellness Journey

FROM PAIN TO WELLNESS:
Overcoming Autoimmune Diseases, An Undisclosed Epidemic

MY JOURNEY TO RECOVERY THROUGH FOOD, LIFESTYLE CHANGES AND SUPPLEMENTS

Ionelia Silvia Prajescu, Eng., INHC

Copyright © 2024 Ionelia Silvia Prajescu

All rights reserved.

No part of this publication may be reproduced, distributed, or transmitted in totality or in part without prior approval from the author.

DEDICATION

To all who navigate the challenging waters of chronic autoimmune diseases,

This book is dedicated to you. To those who feel overlooked and underserved by the medical system that are meant to heal us. Your resilience in the face of invisibility, your courage when faced with daily battles and your strength in moments of despair are nothing short of heroic. May these pages offer you solace, understanding, and a voice that echoes your own experiences. You are not alone, and your journey matters deeply.

With heartfelt solidarity,

Ionelia Silvia Prajescu

Contents

DEDICATION ....
ACKNOWLEDGMENTS v
DISCLAIMER vii
AUTHOR'S NOTES ix
PART I ....
INTRODUCTION ....
1. WHAT ARE AUTOIMMUNE DISEASES? 1
   1.1 WHY DID I WRITE THIS BOOK? 1
   1.2 WHAT IS AUTOIMMUNE DISEASE? 3
   1.3 HASHIMOTO'S, AUTOIMMUNE GASTRITIS (AIG), PERNICIOUS ANEMIA (PA) AND OTHERS 13
PART II 25
MY JOURNEY AND MY EXPERIENCES 25
   2.1 WHO AM I? MY REAL AND IMAGINARY TROUBLES 27
   2.2 STRESS AS A TRIGGER FOR HEALTH ISSUES 37
      2.2.1 WHAT IS STRESS? 39
      2.2.2 HOW TO MANAGE STRESS 44
   2.3 MY REAL TROUBLES ARE JUST STARTING .. 54
   2.4 IT GETS WORSE BEFORE IT GETS BETTER . 59
   2.5 PRESCRIPTION MEDICATION AS A TRIGGER FOR HEALTH ISSUES 71
      2.5.1 WHY MAN-MADE CHEMICAL MEDICATION IS NOT GOOD 73
      2.5.2 STRATEGY TO STOP TAKING PPIs 78

    2.5.3 WHY DO WE NEED STOMACH ACID?......87

  2.6 FINALLY, IT GETS BETTER..............................**123**

    2.6.1 LABORATORY TESTS..................................135

    2.6.2 PERSONALIZED TREATMENT..................148

PART III...**157**

OUR DAY-TO-DAY POTENTIAL AUTOIMMUNE TRIGGERS...157

  3.1 OUR LIFESTYLE..**159**

    3.1.1 OUR FOOD...160

    3.1.2 CHRONIC STRESS...165

    3.1.3 OUR DIET...166

    3.1.4 EXERCISE (OR BETTER SAID THE LACK OF EXERCISE)...169

    3.1.5 SLEEP...171

  3.2 PRESCRIPTION MEDICATIONS.......................**173**

  3.3 OUR ENVIRONMENT...**177**

    3.3.1 AIR QUALITY..178

    3.3.2 WATER QUALITY...181

    3.3.3 MOLDS..184

  3.4 OUR EVERYDAY CHEMICALS EXPOSURE..**187**

    3.4.1 HOUSEHOLD CLEANING PRODUCTS...187

    3.4.2 SKIN CARE PRODUCTS................................190

    3.4.3 DENTAL AMALGAMS...................................192

CONCLUSION..194

PART IV..197

THE DIET..197

4.1 DIFFERENT FACETS OF HEALTH................. 199

4.2 WHAT IS A DIET?.. 201

4.3 HEALTHY FOOD FOR AUTOIMMUNE DISEASES
.... 211

4.4 FOOD LABELS AND INGREDIENTS.............. 223

REFERENCES..229

AUTHOR BIO 239

ACKNOWLEDGMENTS

To my husband and my children,
This book, while a product of my thoughts and experiences, is a testament of the continuous support and love you have provided me.
To my husband, your steadfast companionship and encouragement have been my anchor.
To my children, your existence gave me the power to fight to provide with a better life.
This journey is not mine alone but ours together. **THANK YOU!**

DISCLAIMER

The information provided in this book is based on my personal experiences and research and is intended for informational purposes only. It is not my intention to provide specific medical advice but rather to provide readers with information to better understand their health and their diagnosed disorders. Since each of us is unique, I urge you to consult with a qualified physician for diagnosis and for answers to your personal questions.

This book is not to be taken as medical advice. Always consult with your physician or a qualified healthcare professional regarding any health concerns and before making any medical or lifestyle changes.

By writing this book I aim to increase awareness about the impact of current eating habits and medication, in particular stomach acid medications, on autoimmune diseases. However, the content herein should not be used as a substitute for professional medical advice, diagnosis, or treatment. It is important to consult with a healthcare provider before starting any new medication or supplement regimen, and never discontinue prescribed medication without medical approval.

The dietary and nutrition advice presented is drawn from my experiences and is for informational purposes only. It is not a replacement for professional nutritional counseling.

Remember, no content in this book should replace direct medical advice from your doctor or other qualified healthcare provider.

By accessing the information in this book, you agree to absolve the author of any responsibility for claims, liabilities, damages, or expenses that may arise from the use of this book, including but not limited to legal fees and costs.

AUTHOR'S NOTES

This book is a vital resource for anyone touched by autoimmune diseases, whether you're directly affected, fearful of developing one, or supporting a loved one through their health journey. It's particularly relevant if:

- You're using antacid medication.
- You've been diagnosed with an autoimmune disease (thyroid Hashimoto's or Graves diseases, Rheumatoid Arthritis, Autoimmune Gastritis…).
- You experience heartburn, indigestion, IBS, IBD, asthma, or allergies.

Chronic diseases are alarmingly widespread, with two-thirds of global deaths attributed to them. Often, individuals live with multiple chronic health conditions, navigating a complex healthcare landscape.

My personal health story with an autoimmune disease began in 2013, with a low blood B12 level after four years on daily Proton Pump Inhibitor (PPI) medication therapy. Despite this, my doctors did not express concern. This lack of concern persisted even in 2016 when I developed Hashimoto's thyroiditis after seven years on PPIs. By 2020, despite long-term use of H2-blockers and PPIs, I was diagnosed with gastritis, which finally triggered my concern. My health was deteriorating despite following all prescribed medical advice and following a healthy diet. Furthermore, the solution for the newly gastritis diagnosis was more PPI prescription.

This led me to question the traditional medical approach to chronic conditions. It seemed to be more about trial-and-error using hard medication, than understanding and treating the underlying causes of my illness. I realized that I needed to understand and address the root causes of my health issues, rather than just masking symptoms with medication.

In late 2020, I decided to take a proactive role in my health journey. I began to educate myself and consult with Dr. Susan Blum MD, a functional medicine doctor renowned for her systematic approach to identifying and treating the root causes of illness. This experience reinforced my belief that knowledge is not just power; it's also the key to health.

Functional Medicine presents a promising alternative for managing chronic diseases. Its patient-centered, integrated approach offers a much-needed contrast to the often fragmented and symptom-focused care in conventional medicine.

"The purpose of a writer is to keep civilization from destroying itself."

Albert Camus

Philosopher, author, dramatist, and journalist

PART I

INTRODUCTION

1. WHAT ARE AUTOIMMUNE DISEASES?

1.1 WHY DID I WRITE THIS BOOK?

To paraphrase "knowledge is power" I can say with conviction knowledge is health.

Autoimmune diseases, even in the 21st century, remain somewhat enigmatic to the medical community. This book is intended to explore my viewpoint, as a patient, born from personal struggles and a deep dive into understanding my symptoms and conditions. Unlike many books often linked to commercial interests, my sole aim is to enlighten people about the critical choices we make in life. Our diet, medication, living environment, and stress levels - all have profound effects on our physical, mental, and spiritual well-being. Our health often pays the price for our wrong choices. Ultimately, the length of time we spend here on Earth is unfortunately shortened and its quality is impacted by the physical pain induced by our diseases.

This book aims to raise awareness about the potential of autoimmune diseases to become a widespread health crisis. Historically, the medical community only acknowledged the existence of these diseases in the mid-20th century. Today, the American Autoimmune Association reports over 100 identified autoimmune diseases affecting millions [1]. On July 1st, 2020, an article published in Harvard Health Publishing highlighted an alarming increase in autoimmune diseases, as evidenced by rising positive antinuclear antibody (ANA) tests. Over only two decades the positive ANA test results had risen from 11% during 1988 – 1991 period, to 11.5% during 1999 – 2004 timeframe and finally to 15.9%

in the 2011 – 2012 (14) [2]. This increase, not explainable by genetic changes alone, points towards lifestyle and environmental factors as key contributors.

1.2 WHAT IS AUTOIMMUNE DISEASE?

Navigating the healthcare system with a chronic illness can be a daunting and often a traumatic journey. The prevalence of chronic diseases has seen a significant rise, with factors like epigenetics and lifestyle playing crucial roles.

According to a survey by the Autoimmune Association, 45% of patients with autoimmune diseases have been labeled as 'chronic complainers'. Such patients frequently encounter dismissal and invalidation in the healthcare system, leaving them feeling hopeless and powerless. The lack of adequate answers, solutions, and hope can lead to prolonged physical, mental, and emotional suffering.

The path to an autoimmune diagnosis is often lengthy and arduous. It can take anywhere from 4 to 10 years, and sometimes involves consulting up to 20 different healthcare professionals. This prolonged period of uncertainty, coupled with debilitating symptoms, fosters fear and a sense of isolation among patients. Furthermore, the frequent dismissal of symptoms by doctors, implying that 'it's all in your head', adds to the trauma, creating what can be described as medical gaslighting.

This difficult experience underscores the need for more empathy, understanding, and patient-centered care in the healthcare system, particularly for those living with chronic illnesses.

So, what exactly is an autoimmune disease? To better grasp this concept, let's consider the role of our immune system. Normally, this system is our body's defender against foreign invaders like viruses and bacteria, attacking and destroying them to keep us healthy. However, in the case of autoimmune diseases, this process goes awry. The immune system begins to mistakenly identify our own body's cells as foreign invaders and attacks them. The specific autoimmune disease we develop depends on which part of the body the immune system targets.

For instance:

- If it attacks the thyroid gland, leading to an underactive thyroid, the condition is known as Hashimoto's disease. In contrast, an overactive thyroid caused by immune attack is known as Graves' disease.
- When the stomach lining is the target, it results in Autoimmune Gastritis.
- An attack on the liver leads to Autoimmune Hepatitis.

In fact, nearly any body part can be affected by autoimmune processes.

Many people, as I was in 2016, remain unaware of their autoimmune condition and the doctors do not educate us, the patients, what to do when we develop one, other than taking hard medication to mask the symptoms. This lack of awareness is concerning because, despite their diversity, most autoimmune diseases share common factors. They can be triggered by infections, stress, or certain medications, leading to chronic inflammation which may eventually manifest as an autoimmune disease.

Here is a brief list of some known autoimmune diseases for reference [3]:

- Addison disease: Adrenal glands don't produce enough hormones.
- Celiac disease: Gluten reaction damages the lining of the small intestine.
- Graves disease: Immune system attacks the thyroid, causing hyperthyroidism.
- Hashimoto disease: Immune system attacks the thyroid, leading to hypothyroidism.
- Multiple sclerosis: Attack on the central nervous system (brain and spinal cord).
- Myasthenia gravis: Damage to muscles and the nerves controlling them.

- Pernicious anemia: Vitamin B12 malabsorption leading to a decrease in red blood cells.

- Reactive arthritis: Arthritis symptoms after an infection.

- Rheumatoid arthritis: Inflammation of joints and surrounding tissues.

- Sjogren syndrome: Destruction of glands producing saliva and tears.

- Systemic lupus erythematosus: Attacks healthy tissue such as skin, joints, kidneys, brain.

- Type 1 diabetes: The pancreas produces little or no insulin.

- Inflammatory bowel disease: Attacks the intestines' lining.

- Guillain-Barre syndrome: Attacks nerves controlling muscles.

- Psoriasis: Accelerates skin cell reproduction, leading to skin plaques.

- Chronic inflammatory demyelinating polyneuropathy: Attacks nerves.

- Vasculitis: Damages blood vessels, affecting various organs.

- Autoimmune pancreatitis: Attacks the pancreas and possibly other organs.

- Rheumatic fever: Affects the heart, joints, brain, and skin.

- Vitiligo: Attacks skin cells that produce melanin.

For a more comprehensive list of autoimmune diseases, the Global Autoimmune Institute is a valuable resource [3].

An autoimmune disease fundamentally alters an organ's function. In my case, my stomach stopped producing acid, leading to severe consequences if not properly managed. These diseases occur when the immune system, which typically defends against harmful invaders, mistakenly attacks our own tissues. This can lead to tissue destruction, abnormal growths (tumors), which may be benign or malignant.

Understanding what triggers an autoimmune disease remains a challenge. Genetics play a role; a family history of autoimmune diseases can increase your risk. Other potential triggers include viruses, chemicals, medications, stress, and diet. These factors can contribute to inflammation, making our bodies more susceptible to autoimmune diseases. Personally, I believe that stress and nutrition are very important factors in altering our gut microbiota producing inflammation in our bodies which in turn, when a favorable condition is met, make our body more predisposed to autoimmune diseases.

A common pattern with autoimmune diseases is that developing one often leads to developing others. Hence, early awareness and management of inflammation are crucial. I wish my doctors had emphasized this when I was diagnosed with Hashimoto's in 2016, or, even better, when my B12 levels were low in 2013. An earlier intervention could have potentially altered the course of my autoimmune conditions. I would have completely changed my lifestyle, my diet and hopefully, I could have reversed my B12 deficiency or even Hashimoto without any hard medication and I might have avoided developing the autoimmune gastritis. I wish I knew then what I know now. This book aims to share my experiences, hoping to help others avoid similar struggles.

Autoimmune diseases are chronic, meaning they are long-term conditions. While currently incurable, their symptoms can be managed, and progression can be slowed or halted. Most share a common feature: inflammation. Many times, lifestyle and dietary changes can significantly control this inflammation. In a lot of cases, we can control the inflammation by changing our diet and our lifestyle. In other cases, unfortunately, we need to take medication. However, understanding the side effects of medications and questioning their necessity is very important. Often, doctors, constrained by time and training, focus on symptoms rather than underlying causes, leading to a cycle of medication without addressing the root of the problem. Moreover, the prescribed medication creates other health issues that require other medication and so on and so forth. It becomes a vicious circle.

Diagnosing autoimmune diseases can be notably challenging, and this is especially true for autoimmune gastritis. Typically, when patients present with symptoms indicative of stomach inflammation, gastroenterologists often rely on endoscopy for diagnosis and commonly prescribe proton pump inhibitors (PPIs) as a treatment. However, this approach might not be suitable for autoimmune gastritis. In this condition, the immune system attacks the stomach's parietal cells, which leads to reduced or absent stomach acid production, contrary to the excess acid production seen in other forms of gastritis.

To accurately diagnose autoimmune gastritis, specific tests are necessary. These include blood tests for parietal cell antibodies, intrinsic factor antibodies, and serum gastrin levels. Such specific diagnostic measures are not always a part of routine gastroenterological assessments, leading to potential misdiagnosis or delays in identifying the autoimmune nature of the condition.

The challenge is compounded by the fact that some doctors, particularly those less experienced with autoimmune disorders, may not recognize the distinct characteristics of the stomach lining affected by autoimmune gastritis. Therefore, they might resort to prescribing PPIs based on the observed inflammation, without considering an autoimmune cause. This approach can be problematic since stomach acid, whose production is impaired in autoimmune gastritis, plays a vital role in digesting and assimilating nutrients and maintaining a healthy immune system. Misdiagnosing and treating autoimmune gastritis as a typical acid-related gastritis can therefore overlook these critical aspects of patient health.

In conclusion, a high degree of clinical suspicion and the application of specific tests beyond standard procedures are essential for the accurate diagnosis of an autoimmune disease. Healthcare providers should consider autoimmune causes in patients with persistent gastrointestinal symptoms, especially when conventional treatments are ineffective.

"Recent studies of medical errors have estimated errors may account for as many as 251,000 deaths annually in the United States (U.S), making medical errors the third leading cause of death. Error rates are significantly higher in the U.S. than in other developed countries such as Canada, Australia, Germany and United Kingdom (U.K). At the same time less than 10 percent of medical errors are reported." [4]

The above study does not even take into consideration the diagnostic errors that lead to medication prescriptions that lead to autoimmune diseases that, in turn, lead to premature deaths.

Here are some of the limitations of the current medical system that I identified:

Working in silos: One of the challenges I've observed in the current medical system is the limited communication between different medical specialties. For example, a gastroenterologist (GI doctor) may not always coordinate with an ear, nose, and throat (ENT) doctor, leading to a situation where each specialist treats a specific issue in isolation. This approach can be likened to treating the body as a machine with independent parts, rather than as an interconnected whole.

This lack of integrated care often results in patients being shuffled from one specialist to another. Such fragmentation not only leads to increased time spent in doctors' offices and higher medical expenses but can also cause frustration for patients. More concerning is the risk of being prescribed multiple medications by different specialists, which might not address the underlying health issues effectively and could potentially lead to adverse effects.

However, it's important to recognize that this issue is part of broader systemic challenges in healthcare. These include administrative burdens, time constraints, and resource limitations. While individual healthcare professionals often strive to provide the best care, the structure of the healthcare system can sometimes hinder comprehensive, coordinated treatment.

This system appears particularly ill-equipped to effectively manage chronic conditions, including autoimmune diseases. In my view, there should be a 'marriage' between allopathic (conventional) medicine and functional medicine. Such an integration would acknowledge that we are unique individuals with varying genetic, environmental, dietary, and psychological factors influencing our health. As patients, we must advocate for our health and seek multiple opinions when necessary.

I disagree with the notion that patients should not research their conditions. Understanding our health is crucial, as we know our bodies and minds better than anyone else. While I do not advocate for avoiding necessary medication, being well-informed about potential side effects and the necessity of prescribed treatments is important.

As mentioned previously, the ideal healthcare system would combine the scientific approaches of both allopathic and functional medicine. If considering functional medicine, I recommend consulting a licensed MD who is also certified in functional medicine.

While general practitioners (GPs) are supposed to integrate information from all specialists, in practice, I have found this to be lacking. The feedback and coordination necessary to view a patient's health holistically are often missing. It's like a dysfunctional company where departments work towards their individual goals without aligning with the organization's overall objective – in this case, the patient's well-being. This 'Human Health Company' desperately needs a competent 'CEO,' a role I found, unfortunately, fulfilled only by a good functional medicine doctor.

Continuing Medical Education training for doctors: Another issue I've observed is related to Continuing Medical Education (CME) for doctors. According to cmelist.com/state-cme-requirements/in most states, doctors are required to complete a minimum of 20 credits of CME annually (Florida, Georgia, Hawaii, Idaho, Louisiana, Mississippi, Nevada and others – 40 credits every two years, Kentucky – 60 credits every three years while Indiana, Montana, South Dakota and other states have no CME requirements for physicians) to renew their medical license. These often include conferences and CME programs, many of which are sponsored by pharmaceutical companies. There's a concern that this sponsorship could influence doctors toward prescribing certain medications.

It's essential for medical professionals to stay updated with the latest advancements in their fields by regularly reading medical journals and papers. However, there seems to be a gap in embracing some time-tested medical practices. For instance, comprehensive diagnostic approaches like stool testing for gastrointestinal issues are sometimes overlooked in favor of more straightforward diagnoses like IBS (Irritable Bowel Syndrome). Additionally, the quick attribution of symptoms like abdominal pain and bloating to medications like PPIs (Proton Pump Inhibitors), without deeper investigation, can be problematic.

Since long-term use of antacid medication can alter the gut microbiome [5] and considering that a significant part of our immune system is located in the gut, it's crucial for individuals with a history of extended antacid use to focus on improving and maintaining gut health. Given the vital role of the gut microbiome in both preventing infections and potentially influencing the development of autoimmune diseases, conducting a comprehensive stool test can be a key step in assessing and managing gut health. This approach is particularly important for those who have relied heavily on antacids, as it helps in understanding and addressing any imbalances in the gut flora.

In my experience, consulting a functional medicine doctor for autoimmune diseases or for any disease, has been beneficial. This approach contrasts with some of the skepticism I've encountered from practitioners of conventional medicine regarding functional medicine. Functional medicine often prioritizes lifestyle interventions such as exercise, stress reduction, and diet modifications as primary treatments, which I believe should be more widely adopted in general medical practice. The question I asked myself: why has conventional medicine leaned more towards prescribing medications over these holistic approaches? Talking with people around me I realized that there's a perception that it's simpler for patients to take a pill to alleviate symptoms, and this approach aligns with the interests of pharmaceutical companies, which heavily promote their products.

In my view, the optimal treatment for autoimmune diseases, and health issues in general, lies in a balanced approach that combines the rigor of allopathic medicine with the holistic perspective of functional medicine. Both have their strengths, and when used in conjunction, they can offer a more comprehensive and effective treatment strategy.

Nutrition education offered in the medical school: As of recent data, only 27% of US medical schools offer the recommended 25 hours of nutritional training [22]. On average, medical schools in the United States provide only about 19.6 hours of nutrition education across the entire four-year medical education program. This amount of nutrition education corresponds to less than 1% of the estimated total lecture hours.

Medical insurance: In this final commentary on allopathic versus functional, integrative medicine, I address a critical gap in healthcare coverage. To my knowledge, most insurance plans do not include functional medicine practitioners in their networks. This situation puzzles me, considering the potential long-term benefits of functional medicine. While allopathic doctors, limited by time constraints, may spend about 15 to 30 minutes per patient visit, focusing mainly on symptoms, this approach can lead to short-term cost savings for insurance companies but might not be the most effective strategy in the long run.

Let me elaborate on this point:

Allopathic Medicine: Typically involves brief visits, where the primary focus is on symptom management, often through medication. While this can provide immediate relief, it doesn't always address the root cause of a health issue. The side effects of medications can lead to further health complications, potentially creating a cycle of dependency on drugs.

Functional Medicine: These consultations are more extensive, ranging from 2-3 hours for initial visits to 1-1.5 hours for follow-ups. Functional medicine goes in details into a patient's history, lifestyle, and overall health to identify the root causes of illness. It emphasizes educating patients on healthy living, stress management, and dietary changes aimed at resolving or mitigating health issues.

I firmly believe that a combination of allopathic and functional medicine could provide the most comprehensive care, potentially leading to a healthier, longer life for patients. My personal experiences have inclined me towards functional medicine, and I consider myself a testament to its effectiveness. Changing lifelong habits can be challenging, especially without immediate health concerns as a motivator. Our current lifestyle, characterized by convenience and easy access to unhealthy food options, doesn't always encourage the healthiest choices.

In the following sections, I'll explore key factors influencing our health and the development of autoimmune diseases. Part II of this book will detail my experiences, including insights gained in hindsight about the development of my autoimmune disease, the steps I took, and what could have been done differently.

Part III will discuss various diets. I will add to this book a table with the ingredients allowed by different diets, and I will explain how to use it.

Part IV will offer recipes and tips for creating healthy meals. This resource is aimed at empowering readers to make informed choices for their health and well-being.

Before jumping to the next chapter, I would like to say a few words about Hashimoto's and Autoimmune Gastritis.

1.3 HASHIMOTO'S, AUTOIMMUNE GASTRITIS (AIG), PERNICIOUS ANEMIA (PA) AND OTHERS

Hashimoto's thyroiditis is an autoimmune condition where the immune system attacks the thyroid gland, causing inflammation. This often results in hypothyroidism, characterized by the thyroid's inability to produce enough hormones. The disease is notably more prevalent in women, particularly in white women aged between 40 and 60 years.

The exact causes of Hashimoto's are not fully understood, but it's believed to be a combination of genetic predisposition and environmental factors. Having another autoimmune disease increases the risk of developing Hashimoto's.

Conventional medical treatment typically involves lifelong thyroid hormone replacement to normalize thyroid hormone levels and alleviate symptoms. However, approaches to treatment can vary. Some doctors may delay medication if thyroid hormone levels are within normal ranges, even with elevated thyroid antibodies. In such cases, I believe a dietary approach focusing on reducing inflammation, coupled with monitoring essential minerals and vitamins like B12, D, copper, zinc, iron, selenium, and magnesium, can be beneficial. Unfortunately, this holistic approach isn't always followed, leaving some patients feeling untreated and distressed. On the other hand, some practitioners may quickly resort to lifelong medication, which has its implications for thyroid function over time.

Managing Hashimoto's thyroiditis requires a nuanced approach that considers both the hormonal levels and the patient's overall well-being, including dietary and lifestyle factors. Through my extensive reading and research, I've come to understand the significant impact that Hashimoto's thyroiditis and the resulting hypothyroidism can have on the entire body. This small, butterfly-shaped organ, when not functioning properly, can contribute to a wide array of health issues such as metabolic slowdown leading to reduced energy, fatigue; mental health manifested like depression, anxiety, irritability and difficulties with focus and concentration; cardiovascular risk given by increased risk of elevated cholesterol; digestive issues; musculoskeletal discomfort like joint pain; reproductive issues; dermatological problems affecting the skin and hair, leading to dryness, brittle nails, and hair thinning.

Understanding the broad scope of hypothyroidism's impact stresses, the importance of proper thyroid function and the need for comprehensive management of this condition.

It is my understanding that a thyroid dysfunction negatively affects other organs in our body and to say that - "your thyroid antibodies are not high enough for you to take thyroid medication. I have patients that have TPO higher than 1000, yours at only 167 is not high enough yet" - despite feeling miserable, and without giving any advice to change the diet and lifestyle, is a very narrow view of the situation and shows how little understanding some of our doctors have of the way our body functions as a whole. Luckily, there are more and more studies on how the dysfunction of one part of our body affects the whole body. Unluckily, those studies do not make it to the procedures our doctors are required to follow.

Thyroid dysfunction can potentially affect various organs and systems in the body due to the widespread influence of thyroid hormones. Thyroid hormones play a crucial role in regulating metabolism and energy production, and they have an impact on many physiological processes.

Thyroid disorders and liver - Recent studies have been exploring the connection between thyroid disorders, particularly hypothyroidism, and liver health. There's emerging evidence to suggest a link between Hashimoto's thyroiditis, an autoimmune condition affecting the thyroid gland, and non-alcoholic fatty liver disease (NAFLD) – a condition characterized by excess fat accumulation in the liver not caused by alcohol consumption [6].

A notable 2017 study published in the Journal of Hepatology [7] delved into this association. It found that individuals with higher levels of thyroid peroxidase (TPO) antibodies, commonly elevated in Hashimoto's thyroiditis, had an increased risk of developing NAFLD. This finding is significant as it sheds light on the broader systemic effects of thyroid disorders.

Furthermore, a review in the World Journal of Hepatology emphasized the potential roles of insulin resistance, inflammation, and oxidative stress in both Hashimoto's thyroiditis and NAFLD. These shared factors suggest that the two conditions may be linked through common biological pathways.

Thyroid disorders and kidneys - The study titled 'Thyroid dysfunction and kidney disease: An update,' published in 2017 in 'Reviews in Endocrine & Metabolic Disorders,' [8] delves into the relationship between thyroid disorders and kidney function. It particularly highlights the impact conditions like Hashimoto's thyroiditis can have on the kidneys.

Thyroid hormones are known to influence renal development, glomerular filtration rate (GFR), and electrolyte homeostasis. Thus, thyroid dysfunctions, including both hypothyroidism and hyperthyroidism, can lead to various renal complications. In hypothyroidism, for instance, reduced thyroid hormone levels can lead to decreased kidney function, as indicated by lower GFR rates. Conversely, hyperthyroidism can cause an increase in GFR, potentially leading to other renal issues.

The study emphasizes the importance of regular kidney function monitoring in patients with thyroid disorders. This is particularly crucial as changes in thyroid function can subtly yet significantly alter kidney function. Early detection and management of these changes can prevent further complications and ensure better overall management of both thyroid and kidney health.

Moreover, the study underlines the bidirectional nature of this relationship, as not only can thyroid dysfunction affect kidney health, but kidney disease can also have implications for thyroid function. This two-way relationship necessitates a comprehensive approach to patient care, where management of one condition incorporates considerations for the potential impact on the other.

Thyroid disorders and brain and nervous system: In infants and children, congenital hypothyroidism, if left untreated, can have serious consequences, leading to intellectual disabilities and developmental delays [9]. Early detection and treatment are critical to prevent these irreversible effects.

In adults, thyroid disorders impact the nervous system differently [10]. Hypothyroidism can lead to neurological symptoms, including cognitive impairment and mood alterations. Patients might experience difficulties with memory, slowed thinking, depression, and an overall sense of lethargy. On the other hand, hyperthyroidism, particularly in cases like Graves' disease, can manifest as nervousness, anxiety, and mood swings.

Additionally, hyperthyroidism, especially related to Graves' disease, can affect the eyes [11]. Patients may experience symptoms like double vision, though more common symptoms include eye bulging, redness, and irritation.

Thyroid disorders and cardiovascular system: Thyroid hormones play a crucial role in regulating the cardiovascular system, influencing heart rate, blood pressure, and the strength of heart muscle contractions [12]. In cases of hyperthyroidism, where there is an excess of thyroid hormones, individuals often experience an increased heart rate, palpitations, and higher blood pressure. These symptoms are due to the thyroid hormones stimulating the heart to beat faster and more forcefully.

Conversely, hypothyroidism, characterized by insufficient thyroid hormone production, can lead to a reduced heart rate. This slowdown in cardiac activity can be accompanied by an increase in cholesterol levels, which is a notable risk factor for heart disease. The reduced metabolic rate associated with hypothyroidism contributes to this altered lipid profile, underscoring the importance of thyroid function in cardiovascular health.

Therefore, both hyperthyroidism and hypothyroidism present distinct challenges to the cardiovascular system. Hyperthyroidism primarily causes the heart to work harder and faster, whereas hypothyroidism can lead to a slower heart function and altered lipid metabolism, both of which can significantly impact overall heart health.

Thyroid disorders and reproductive system: Thyroid disorders can have a significant impact on the reproductive system [13]. In women, imbalances in thyroid hormones can disrupt menstrual regularity, leading to irregular or missed periods. This disruption can extend to fertility, as normal thyroid function is essential for regular ovulation and reproductive health.

In both men and women, thyroid dysfunction can also influence libido and overall sexual function. Hypothyroidism, for example, can lead to a decreased sex drive, while hyperthyroidism might cause an increased libido but could also be associated with another sexual dysfunction.

The effects of thyroid hormones on reproductive health are multifaceted, affecting everything from menstrual cycle regularity to sexual desire and performance. Given the thyroid's integral role in regulating hormones, any dysfunction in this gland can lead to a cascade of changes in the reproductive system.

Thyroid disorders and musculoskeletal system: Thyroid hormones play an integral role in the health of the musculoskeletal system [14]. They are vital for the proper metabolism of bones and the maintenance of muscle mass, ensuring both strength and mobility.

In the context of thyroid dysfunction, particularly hypothyroidism, there can be significant musculoskeletal consequences. Untreated hypothyroidism often leads to muscle weakness, which can manifest as a general feeling of fatigue or specific muscle aches. Patients may also experience joint pain, adding to discomfort and potentially impacting daily activities.

The impact on bone metabolism in hypothyroidism can also be notable. While hyperthyroidism is more commonly associated with accelerated bone loss and increased fracture risk, hypothyroidism, especially when severe and untreated, can also affect bone density and health, albeit in a different mechanism.

Thyroid disorders and digestive system: Thyroid hormones significantly influence the digestive system, particularly in regulating how quickly food moves through the gastrointestinal tract. In cases of hypothyroidism, where thyroid hormone levels are low, this can lead to a slowdown in gut motility [15]. Consequently, individuals with hypothyroidism often experience constipation, a direct result of this reduced gastrointestinal movement.

On the other hand, hyperthyroidism, characterized by excessive thyroid hormone production, can lead to increased gut motility. This heightened activity can manifest as diarrhea, reflecting the overall accelerated metabolic processes in the body.

This modification of gut's motility associated with hypothyroidism could predispose to small intestinal bacterial overgrowth which may lead to gut impermeability also known as "leaky gut", which in turn can lead to other autoimmune diseases [16].

Beyond these direct effects on gut motility, there's emerging evidence suggesting a potential link between thyroid dysfunction and gallbladder health. Specifically, hypothyroidism has been associated with an increased risk of gallstones. This association is thought to arise from decreased gallbladder motility and altered bile composition in individuals with underactive thyroid function.

Thyroid disorders and cholecystectomy: A study published in 2018 [17] sheds light on the broader implications of Hashimoto's thyroiditis, revealing a notable association with an increased rate of cholecystectomy, the surgical removal of the gallbladder. This finding is significant as it underscores the diverse impacts of Hashimoto's beyond the thyroid gland itself.

Interestingly, this increased rate of gallbladder surgery was observed in patients with Hashimoto's regardless of whether they were receiving thyroxine treatment. This suggests that the autoimmune nature of Hashimoto's, which involves chronic inflammation and immune system dysregulation, might contribute to gallbladder issues independently of thyroid hormone levels. It implies that even with thyroid hormone levels managed through medication, patients with Hashimoto's might still be at an elevated risk for gallbladder problems.

This echoes my personal experience in 2020, four years after being diagnosed with Hashimoto's, when I had to undergo gallbladder removal because it was no longer releasing the bile. Regrettably, my gastroenterologist and GI surgeon were unable to provide an explanation for why my gallbladder ceased to function, leading me to the conclusion that they lack understanding of the connection between Hashimoto's and gallbladder malfunction. The study above indicates that monitoring and managing potential gallbladder issues should be an integral part of the overall treatment plan, even for those patients who are on thyroxine replacement therapy. Understanding these associations can lead to more proactive and preventive healthcare strategies for patients with Hashimoto's, potentially reducing the risk of complications that could necessitate surgical interventions like cholecystectomy.

I enumerated above the impact that a thyroid that does not function properly can have on our body. In discussing the treatment of thyroid disorders, particularly Hashimoto's thyroiditis, it's evident that the most common approach in conventional medicine is the prescription of Levothyroxine, a synthetic form of the thyroid hormone thyroxine (T4). This treatment is typically based on thyroid function tests, which measure T4 and thyroid-stimulating hormone (TSH) levels. However, this approach often focuses on symptom management rather than addressing the autoimmune root cause of the thyroid's reduced hormone production. Testing for minerals (Selenium, Iron, Copper, Zinc), vitamins (D, B12, B2) and discussions about your diet are not even considered as part of a treatment for thyroid disease.

There is a strong relationship between hypothyroidism and poor absorption of nutrients due to a poor digestion which continues to aggravate the hypothyroidism. I heard a lot of people with Hashimoto's complaining about their endocrinologists not willing to test for minerals and vitamins saying that "they never heard of such a thing". Vitamin B12 deficiency is more common in individuals with Hashimoto's. Stomach acid (intrinsic factor) is essential for the absorption of vitamin B12 from food and having low stomach acid can impair the absorption of other essential nutrients such as iron, calcium, magnesium, copper, zinc and certain vitamins. There is a strong link between gut dysbiosis and thyroid function. According to a study published in 2020 [18], imbalances in the gut microbiome damage the intestinal bacteria increasing the intestinal permeability which can impact the thyroid function.

Thyroid and intestinal diseases coexist, thyroid imbalances affecting the gut health and the gut microbiome composition and intestinal permeability by its capability of absorbing the vitamins and minerals necessary to an optimal thyroid function is impacting the thyroid health creating this way a vicious circle. This connection between the thyroid and the gut is known as the thyroid-gut axis and has led to studies on how the microbiota is influencing the absorption of minerals such as iodine, selenium, zinc, copper and iron to support the thyroid function.

Despite hormone replacement therapy, many individuals with Hashimoto's continue to experience a range of symptoms, impacting their quality of life. Symptoms like fatigue, insomnia, and mental fog can persist, signifying the need for a more comprehensive treatment strategy.

Addressing these concerns involves more than just medication; it requires a multifaceted approach that considers dietary changes, lifestyle modifications, and possibly supplements to address deficiencies. Effective management of Hashimoto's thyroiditis calls for patient-centered care. This approach involves open communication between patient and healthcare provider, where symptoms, treatment responses, and lifestyle factors are thoroughly discussed.

Empowering patients with education about their condition, dietary recommendations, and lifestyle adjustments can lead to more effective management of Hashimoto's and improve overall quality of life.

The thyroid function is very complex, and its hormones affect every cell of our body. It is a very interesting read and, if you suffer from a thyroid dysfunction, I strongly suggest getting books that describe its role and the importance of minerals and vitamins for a good functioning of the thyroid. In addition, controlling the stress in your life, a balanced diet and lifestyle are crucial in keeping the thyroid dysfunction under control, and the most important thing is to be informed and to advocate for yourself.

Autoimmune gastritis (AIG) is an autoimmune disorder in which the immune system mistakenly attacks and damages the cells of the stomach lining, particularly the parietal cells and chief cells which leads to a reduction in stomach acid production and intrinsic factor. As a result, the stomach lining becomes inflamed and undergoes atrophic changes, leading to thinning of the mucosal layer and the development of intestinal metaplasia, where the normal stomach lining cells are replaced by cells similar to those found in the intestines.

Like any other autoimmune disease, the causes of the AIG are not completely understood but it is thought that genetic predisposition and environmental triggers may play an important role. As we now know that the genetic predisposition controls only 10% of our health, it means that the environmental exposure and lifestyle controls the rest of 90%. Latest research suggests that alterations in the gut microbiome may influence the development of autoimmune diseases and we also know that AIG is often associated with other autoimmune diseases, in particular with Hashimoto's thyroiditis and type 1 diabetes [19, 20, 21]. Some studies have suggested a potential link between long-term use of PPIs and an increased risk of autoimmune gastritis. A systematic review and meta-analysis done in 2014 found no "clear" evidence that long-term PPI can cause gastric atrophy or intestinal metaplasia, "although the results were imprecise". The author notes in his conclusions that "People with PPI maintenance treatment may have higher possibility of experiencing either diffuse (simple) or linear/micronodular (focal) enterochromaffin-lice (ECL) hyperplasia" [22]. Three years later, in 2017, another study found evidence that gastric atrophy was statistically higher in those taking PPIs [23].

Autoimmune gastritis is considered a relatively rare condition and for this reason, it may be underdiagnosed or misdiagnosed as other gastric conditions, especially gastritis and most of the time prescribed PPIs. The Proton Pump Inhibitor (PPI) medication is lowering even more the stomach acid which leads to even more mineral and vitamin deficiencies and intestinal dysbiosis which in turn leads to chronic inflammation, immune system dysfunction and mental health through the gut-brain axis connection.

Autoimmune gastritis should be diagnosed through a combination of medical history, physical examination blood tests and diagnostic procedures. Blood tests are a crucial component of the diagnostic process for AIG and the following tests should be ordered:

- Complete Blood Count (CBC) to check for anemia or other blood abnormalities.

- Vitamin B12 levels which may indicate a problem with the intrinsic factor absorption.

- Gastrin levels which may suggest reduced stomach acid production if the levels are high.

- Antibody tests such as anti-parietal cell antibodies and anti-intrinsic factor antibodies.

As I mentioned previously, since this is a disease that can be easily misdiagnosed you have to be your own advocate and ask for the above tests if you suspect you have AIG (high levels of anti-parietal cell antibodies, low levels of vitamins D and B12).

An upper endoscopy with biopsy will confirm if there are any characteristic changes, such as atrophy and metaplasia which are indicative of autoimmune gastritis. It is important to note that there is no specific "current protocol" uniformly used by all GI doctors in the United States. The location of the biopsies during an upper endoscopy may vary among different healthcare institutions, individual GI doctors and pathologists. Factors that may influence the selection of a specific protocol or guidelines for histological evaluation include local practices, institutional preferences and individual expertise. Despite the fact that in 1990 was developed the Sydney protocol some medical centers or regions may have developed their own guidelines or adaptations of the Sydney protocol to better suit their specific clinical needs.

The Sydney protocol was developed during the Sydney International Workshop on the Classification of Gastritis in 1990 and has become a widely adopted method in pathology practice. It provides standardized guidelines for the histological evaluation of gastric biopsies taken during an upper endoscopy procedure. Its value is in providing consistent and reproducible diagnoses and it allows for the classification of various types of gastritis, including chronic gastritis, active gastritis, and specific patterns associated with Helicobacter pylori infection. It also helps in identifying precancerous changes, such as atrophy and intestinal metaplasia, which may be associated with an increased risk of gastric cancer.

According to the Sydney protocol, there have to be performed at least five biopsies from four specific areas of the stomach:

1. Antrum: this is the lower part of the stomach, and it assesses changes and inflammation due to Helicobacter pylori
2. Corpus (Body): This is the central part of the stomach, and it helps assess inflammation, atrophy and other histological changes.
3. Incisura Angularis: this is the notch in the lesser curvature of the stomach, and it provides information about Helicobacter pylori infection and inflammation.
4. Greater curvature: It helps assess overall gastric health and identify histological changes.

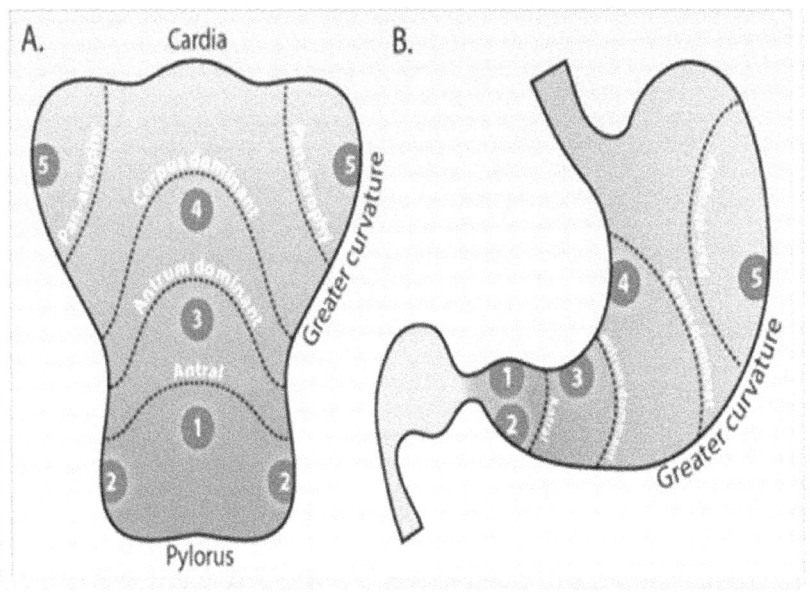

From the paper "British Society of Gastroenterology guidelines on the diagnosis and management of patients at risk of gastric adenocarcinoma" (https://gut.bmj.com/content/gutjnl/early/2019/07/05/gutjnl-2018-318126.full.pdf)

According to a paper published in 2020 [24], there is a need to standardize the upper endoscopy practices to help in the diagnosis and the evolution of gastric changes. Several papers [25] mention the importance of using an updated Sydney protocol to improve the diagnostic yield of gastric diagnosis and early detection of chronic atrophic gastritis and autoimmune gastritis.

Since none of the GI doctors I have consulted up to now does use the Sydney protocol in performing the biopsies it is up to us, the patients, to demand the GI doctor performing the endoscopy to follow a systematic approach in executing the biopsies. This is important for making sure the places where the biopsies are taken are repetitive to detect any change of the stomach lining from one procedure to the next.

PART II

MY JOURNEY AND MY EXPERIENCES

2.1 WHO AM I? MY REAL AND IMAGINARY TROUBLES

"When I look back on all these worries, I remember the story of the old man who said on his deathbed that he had had a lot of trouble in his life, most of which had never happened."

Winston Churchill

It all started in November 1993, when I immigrated from Romania to Canada with my husband and our two children, a daughter seven years old and a boy five years old. My husband and I were (and still are) both mechanical engineers trying to find a better life for ourselves but more importantly, to offer a brighter future to our children. Due to the unfavorable exchange rate at that time between the Romanian Leu and the US Dollar, to be able to buy plane tickets for us four, we had to sell our apartment (a four-bedroom-two-baths condo in Bucharest), the car and some furniture. After buying the plane tickets, we were left with $2,000 that we deposited in a bank in Montreal. The idea was to keep this money available for return plane tickets in case we would not succeed in making a better life and wanted to return to our native country. We were determined to make it work though, despite the fear of the unknown and, so we did.

If you have never been in a situation to leave your country, your family, your friends and start an adventure with a lot of unknown, you might not understand the experience and what an immigrant goes through. Even amongst us, the immigrants, the experience is different, the way each of us reacts to each experience we go through is different. Add to this the fact that we each have a different stress threshold and you will find the recipe for stress-induced illnesses. Some people come to friends or family in the new country, some others receive assistance from their church either in form of housing, clothing, advice or even jobs. Some people come directly hired by a company in their new country, some others come with a lot of money, while others come with perfectly mastered languages. Neither of those were true in our case. We landed in Montreal on a cold winter night with no jobs, no house, poorly mastered French and English, worried of what the future holds for us but full of hopes that everything will be alright.

When we landed in Montreal, Canada was getting out of one of its biggest recessions (1990 – 1992) classified as category 4 (recessions are classified from 1 to 5, 1 having a mild impact on unemployment and 5 having an important impact and for a long period of time) and my husband and I were competing against more than 5,000 unemployed engineers, most of them trained in North American universities.

I will not go into the details of how I found employment almost a year after our arrival and after going into tens of interviews for different positions: as engineer I did not have Canadian experience (whatever that meant), as draftsperson or lab technician I was too qualified. Suffice to say that, finally, I got a job as a contractor design engineer for a major company in Montreal but paid less than a technician. In my opinion, that first job was a win-win situation: while the company got a high qualified person for a very low salary, I got my foot through the Canadian workforce door, acquiring Canadian experience and opening the opportunities for my future, advancing almost every 2-3 years in higher and higher positions.

Without even realizing it, the stress started to build up. I was not prepared for my new reality:

There (in Romania) I was coming from a communist country where every person had a job secured for life, from the moment you finished school to the moment you retire. There, we did not even need to write a Resume (Curriculum Vitae) since changing jobs was not an option.

Here (in North America), being hired as a contractor without any benefits, vacation, or sick days, established the foundation on which the stress started to build its walls and make a house in my life.

There, we had both a steady, secure job.

Here, for a couple of years I was the only breadwinner in the family. Living on government welfare was not an option for us.

There, I was talking in my maternal tongue.

Here, I was not very proficient at the beginning neither in French nor in English. My foreign languages skills were based on what I learned in school so, at work, during the meetings, I was understanding a little less than half of what was being discussed, the rest of it I was guessing. It looks like my guess was correct though since everybody was very happy with my work performance. But all these added a brick after another on my stress wall that was building around and inside me.

Stress, a complex and multifaceted phenomenon, can present itself in various forms. Sometimes it appears as a strong, unmistakable emotion following an unpleasant experience, making it easily recognizable. In such cases, one can promptly take steps to mitigate its impact on health. However, stress can also insidiously seep into our lives, often going unnoticed until its effects become too significant to ignore. This subtler form of stress was my experience, particularly because I was deeply engaged in my work and thrived on the challenges it presented.

Almost a decade after immersing myself in this new life and career, the physical manifestations of this long-term, accumulated stress began to emerge. The symptoms were severe and specific: intense pain in the upper part of my stomach, right under my breastbone. These episodes of pain were sporadic but recurring, appearing 3-4 times per year and lasting for 2-3 hours at a stretch, spread over a week. There seemed to be no clear trigger or pattern to these flare-ups; they happened at various times – interrupting my day, disturbing my sleep, sometimes before meals, other times after. Despite my efforts to identify a cause, the pattern of these painful episodes remained elusive.

By this stage, I had not only become fluent in French and English but had also carved out a successful career for myself. I had transitioned from being a newcomer struggling with language barriers to a confident professional holding a permanent, stable job.

However, with professional life came its inherent challenges. There were times when a design wouldn't meet the expected standards in tests, or we had to brainstorm alternative solutions to mitigate risks in a project, or strategize to bring delayed schedules back on track. While I found my work occasionally stressful, it was often more challenging and stimulating than distressing.

The idea that stress could be the underlying cause of my physical symptoms did cross my mind from time to time. However, I quickly dismissed this notion for two main reasons:

- Firstly, leaving my job due to stress wasn't a viable option. I was the one in the family with a more stable and crucial job, so the idea of resigning was out of the question.

- Secondly, there was no apparent correlation between the peak moments of my stress and the timing of these painful episodes. They seemed to happen randomly, sometimes during a busy workweek, but also during weekends or even while I was on vacation, a time when I was supposed to be completely relaxed.

Despite these irregularities, my past experiences gradually heightened my sensitivity to the nuanced effects of emotional stress. I endeavored to understand if there was a specific event, physical sensation, or mental state that triggered this pain. Yet, nothing stood out. This uncertainty led me to consult a doctor. However, all the blood tests and medical examinations I underwent came back negative. The pain was vaguely attributed to something I might have eaten, and the possibility of emotional stress being the root cause was quickly dismissed. It was around 2004-2005, a period when the medical community was still skeptical about the idea that mental and emotional stress could manifest in physical ailments. My doctor, like many others at the time, did not entertain the notion that psychological stress could lead to such physical symptoms.

In the absence of medical validation and facing the practical realities of my life, I chose to sideline my suspicions about stress being the culprit. Rather than exploring alternative paths like changing careers, delving into stress-reducing practices such as meditation or breathing exercises, I continued with my life, trying to push aside the pain. I convinced myself to ignore these distressing episodes, treating them as isolated incidents until they recurred. This approach led me to adapt to living with the pain, accepting it as an unwelcome yet enduring part of my life. In doing so, I inadvertently learned a hard lesson about the complex relationship between our mental state and physical health, and how easily one can overlook critical warning signs when they manifest in unexpected ways.

In my life, other than my work, two particularly stressful events stand out. In 2005, a serious health issue within my family triggered my first and only panic attack, leading to a harrowing experience in the emergency room. This episode underscored my profound anxiety about family health crises, especially when I'm not able to offer support. The second major stressor, which used to haunt me but no longer does, was the fear of job loss and the ensuing financial implications for my children's education and activities.

The year 2005 marked also a significant turning point when our company was acquired by a Mexican business. Despite assurances that our work lives would remain unchanged, the new ownership-initiated changes profoundly affected many. Fast forward to 2008, the closure of the Technology Department was announced, with the transfer of product design to Mexico, resulting in over 40 employees, including my husband and myself, being laid off. The closure not only jeopardized our careers but also raised concerns about our ability to financially support our children, who were then in college.

In a twist of fate, out of the many laid-off employees, five (my husband and I included) were offered a two-year contract to move to Mexico and share our expertise with the engineering team there. My husband and I, facing limited job prospects in Montreal and considering our age, decided to accept this offer. This decision was not made lightly. It meant leaving behind our home, our children, my parents (whom we had sponsored to come to Canada in 1995), and our friends. We were embarking on a new adventure, stepping into the unknown, while leaving behind the life we had built and grown accustomed to over the past 15 years.

The decision to move to Mexico was a mix of emotions – excitement for the new adventure and worry about what the future held post-contract. With more than 15 years left until retirement, the prospect of what would come after our stint in Mexico was a source of concern. The move represented not just a physical relocation but a significant life transition, challenging us to adapt once again to a new environment and culture while being mindful of the responsibilities and ties we had back in Canada.

This period of my life stresses (pun intended) the dynamic and often unpredictable nature of stress, shaped by external events and internal concerns.

My tenure in Mexico was a tapestry of both delightful and taxing experiences. On the one hand, the company's generosity was remarkable, offering comprehensive support including housing, utilities, transportation, and even a private Spanish tutor. These provisions made our stay comfortable and allowed us to explore the rich cultural customs of Mexico. Our weekends and holidays were filled with vibrant explorations of Mexican traditions, cuisine, and the warmth of its people. This aspect of our Mexican sojourn was thoroughly enjoyable and deeply enriching.

On the other hand, the professional side of my experience presented its own set of challenges. The primary stressor was the work environment, characterized by high-pressure projects with tight deadlines. We were tasked with managing multiple programs simultaneously and had to guide a new team that lacked experience in our product's design. This not only tested our professional capabilities but also added a significant amount of stress to the entire team. The task of constructing a new laboratory to test units further compounded this stress, creating a challenging and often tense work atmosphere.

Additionally, the language barrier presented a unique challenge. While I am now grateful for the opportunity it provided to learn Spanish authentically, at the time, the necessity to communicate in an unfamiliar language was daunting. Every conversation and message in Spanish was a hurdle, often leading to misunderstandings and frustration. This aspect of my experience, though educational, was fraught with difficulties and added a layer of complexity to my daily professional interactions.

In summary, my time in Mexico was a blend of personal growth, cultural immersion, and professional challenges. It was an experience that, while at times difficult, offered a wealth of learning and development opportunities. The juxtaposition of enjoying the cultural richness of Mexico with the demanding work environment epitomized the dual nature of such international assignments. The experience not only broadened my horizons culturally but also honed my skills in navigating complex professional landscapes and overcoming language barriers. This period of my life stands as a testament to the resilience required in adapting to new environments and the value of embracing both the joys and challenges that come with such transformative experiences.

In the spring of 2009, the now-familiar pain behind my breastbone returned, continuing its annual cycle that started a long time ago. Despite its persistence, I found it hard to accept stress as the underlying cause. I rationalized that the challenges I was facing were normal, a part of life that everyone encounters without necessarily experiencing physical pain. I enjoyed confronting challenges and believed that I had no choice but to continue working, feeling trapped in my situation. Quitting my job would mean not only my unemployment but also my husband's, plunging us into uncertainty upon our return to Montreal. The other option was to continue working and the pain will go away like it did in all the previous years.

A few years back, one of my colleagues mentioned something about H-Pylori, a bacterium that likes acidic environments and lives in our stomach. These bacteria might cause inflammation in the stomach and duodenum in some people and when it does, it is felt as an ache or burning pain in the stomach, amongst other symptoms. To eliminate this potential cause for my pains I decided to go and ask the opinion of a gastroenterologist in a private medical clinic in the city I was living in then, in Mexico.

The resulting diagnosis from an endoscopy was startling: Barrett's Esophagus, a term unfamiliar to me at the time, which is equivalent to a precancerous condition of the esophagus. This was the first time I had an endoscopy but, in my mind, I did not expect the doctor to find anything abnormal. Now, I had a name for what was causing my pain.

The doctor observed a subtle but significant change in the coloration of my esophagus's lining, a shift from its normal pink to a reddish hue, and took biopsies for a more detailed analysis.

While waiting for the biopsy result to come in, I started to search on the internet as much information as I could find about the Barret's Esophagus symptoms, causes and treatment. My findings painted a frightening picture, intensifying my fears to the point where my thoughts were now obsessed with this disease. As expected, the medical community does not know the exact cause of this condition, however, the consensus is that a gastroesophageal reflux disease (GERD) increases the chances of developing it [26]. The interesting fact is that I never had acid reflux, I never had the burning sensation of the acid going up the food pipe called esophagus and my Lower Esophagus Sphincter (LES, the valve between the esophagus and the stomach, which leaves the food go into the stomach but closes to stop the same food going back into the esophagus), was working well and it was not weak. Other than having the above said sharp-cutting pain behind my breastbone around 3-4 times per year, I did not have any other symptoms and I felt quite healthy. It seems though that around half of the people diagnosed with Barret's esophagus do not have symptoms of acid reflux.

According to Mayo Clinic, the risk factors for increasing the risk of developing Barrett's Esophagus are [27]: family history (nobody in my family had esophagus problems), being a male (not a risk for me), being white (this is true in my case but I don't think it's enough for developing it), being over 50 (that year I was turning 50 but the symptoms were now present for about 10 years), chronic heartburn and acid reflux (I never felt the acid reflux hurting my esophagus other than the pain I was feeling in my chest four times per year), current or past smoking (I stopped smoking 10 years earlier after around 20 years of smoking half of pack of cigarettes per day), being overweight (I was not slim but neither overweight at that time). According to the study "Risk factors for Barrett's esophagus: a scoping review", published in PubMed.gov the conclusion is the same as above after studying a sample size that ranged from 68 to 84,606 [28]. Strangely enough, stress doesn't seem to be part of the risk factors according to these studies. However, stress is felt by a lot of women as a cramp in the stomach and it is mentioned in other medical articles as causing "stomach pain and other GI symptoms".

Barrett's Esophagus is associated with an increased risk of developing esophageal cancer and from my readings at that time, this type of cancer is very aggressive with a poor prognosis. Depending on the stage of cancer the life expectancy is not very encouraging with a 5-year survival rate of less than 20%.

My anxiety for my health was now going through the roof. Since I am not an exception to the rule, I also went through different feelings: first I felt overwhelmed by all the news and by all the less than comforting information I could find. Then, I felt the anger, panic and frustration taking control over me. I felt guilt for not seeking more specialized medical advice sooner and the fear of not witnessing my children's milestones and the possibility of a foreshortened future weighed heavily on me.

Determined to take control of my health, I meticulously started to investigate and analyze the options that I had. I found out that besides the periodic surveillance in the form of endoscopies and biopsies, the only other option is to decrease the acid in the stomach using strong medication like Proton Pump Inhibitors (PPIs): Prevacid, Nexium, Prilosec or Protonix. In terms of diet, there were only a few internet sites that mention some foods to avoid: fried and fatty foods, chocolate, mint, alcohol, coffee, carbonated drinks, citrus fruits or juices and vinegar. Very few sites also mentioned sleeping on an inclined surface with the head raised to take advantage of the natural gravity and help the acid and stomach fluids go down towards the small intestine instead of going up towards the esophagus.

A week after my endoscopy, the biopsy result was ready: no intestinal cells found, no metaplasia (no conversion of esophagus cells into intestinal cells) and no dysplasia (no abnormal development of cells or tissue due to a precancerous stage of growth). So, in my free translation, it is not sure if I have or have not Barrett's Esophagus. The doctor was very nice and very polite, and he also strongly advised me to get another doctor's opinion. He gave me the specimen of my biopsy and recommended bringing it to another lab to have a second lab opinion. Meanwhile, he prescribed Nexium, 1 pill of 40 mg each morning, saying that I will have to take it for life if I want to stop the erosion of my esophagus. He also mentioned that there were no known side effects from taking a PPI and that from now on, due to this medication I would not feel, ever, the stabbing pain behind my breastbone. No interest in the stress level in my life, no mention of any diet changes, no advice on how I should improve my lifestyle to prevent future health issues.

I went home trying to make sense of all this. I started to take Nexium, as prescribed, I eliminated from my diet the few items that are known to increase stomach acid (tomatoes, peppers in addition the list I mentioned above), I raised the head of my bed by about 8 inches which caused me some trouble keeping me from sliding down towards the foot of the bed during nighttime and I replaced carbonated drinks with herbal teas like marshmallow root and slippery elm. These herbal teas are known for creating a coating over the mucus membranes of the stomach and the esophagus, providing a relief from the acid reflux (that I still did not feel) and from inflammation of the stomach and food pipe lining.

I was a woman with a plan now and I started to feel better, at least mentally; my anxiety due to my newly discovered health issues dropped to almost zero. These measures brought a sense of empowerment and a significant reduction in my anxiety. I was confident that I had addressed the root cause of my chest pains and that they were now behind me. I could not have been more wrong: the root cause was not addressed by the medication I was prescribed, but only the symptom, with devastating results on my health.

This newfound confidence would soon be tested, as the journey with my medication began to reveal its own set of complexities. My experience with Barrett's Esophagus was becoming a profound lesson in the interconnectedness of physical health, emotional well-being, and the importance of a holistic approach to medical care.

Without knowing, I was entering another phase of my life in which the medication started to take the first stage in affecting my health but before going there, let's take a look at the stress as a trigger for health issues and how to deal with it.

2.2 STRESS AS A TRIGGER FOR HEALTH ISSUES

Even when all is known, the care of a man is not yet complete, because eating alone will not keep a man well; he must also take exercise. For food and exercise, while possessing opposite qualities, yet work together to produce health.

Hippocrates, Greek physician, the Father of Medicine

Two decades ago, the direct link between stress and chronic diseases was not well-supported by scientific studies. My family doctor at the time regretfully informed me of the lack of concrete evidence linking stress to physical health impact. However, in recent years, there has been a significant shift. More studies now highlight the harmful effects of prolonged, chronic stress on our well-being [29].

The 2017 EXCLI Journal article, "The impact of stress on body function: A review," offers a comprehensive analysis of how stress affects various body systems. It details the impact of stress on brain function and complications, memory, cognition, learning, the immune system, cardiovascular health, gastrointestinal complications, and the endocrine system. The article concludes that many disorders originate from stress, particularly when it is severe and prolonged. It underscores the need for the medical community to recognize and treat stress as a contributing factor in various diseases, advocating for a combination of pharmacological (medications and nutraceuticals) and non-pharmacological (lifestyle changes, daily exercise, healthy nutrition, and stress reduction programs) interventions [30].

When under stress, the body releases hormones such as cortisol, cortisone, DHEA, and homocysteine. These hormones can significantly impact the immune system, especially if the stress becomes chronic. Often, people try to compensate for stress by indulging in unhealthy eating habits. This combination of poor diet and stress hormones can create a direct pathway to various diseases, some of which can be life-threatening if not addressed through lifestyle changes.

This evolving understanding of stress and health underscores the importance of holistic approaches to managing stress, recognizing its potential to trigger or exacerbate health issues. It also highlights the critical role of lifestyle choices in mitigating the adverse effects of stress on our bodies.

2.2.1 WHAT IS STRESS?

"We all know that stress has this great control over us, but the fact is that we really have to take it to heart. We really have to believe that it's having an effect on us so that we can take steps to change what's happening. Try to think of it as if we have these 'stress auras' around us, but stress is actually the way our bodies are responding to them, and we do have control over that."

Susan Blum, MD, MPH, Functional Medicine Doctor, and Founder of Blum Center for Health

We hear lately people saying that they are stressed out, but what is stress? According to Merriam-Webster definition, stress is:

1. A force exerted when one body or body part presses on, pulls on, pushes against, or tends to compress or twist another body or body part.
2. The deformation caused in a body by such a force.
3. A physical, chemical, or emotional factor that causes bodily or mental tension and may be a factor in disease causation.
4. A state resulting from stress especially: one of bodily or mental tension resulting from factors that tend to alter an existing equilibrium //job-related stress.
5. strain, pressure.

Stress, as defined by Merriam-Webster, encompasses a range of responses – physical or emotional – to situations that disturb our equilibrium or comfort zone. It encompasses everything from the physical stress of an injury to the mental strain of daily life challenges.

Acute physical stress, such as pulling a muscle or fracturing a limb, is a clear, tangible form of stress. These injuries result in immediate physical discomfort, but typically, the body heals from such trauma within a few weeks. This type of stress is straightforward in both its identification and treatment.

Without any doubt, the most difficult to diagnose despite its important contribution in developing a disease is the emotional stress.

The landscape of emotional stress is far more complex and nuanced. Emotional stress can be real, triggered by immediate, palpable threats to our safety or well-being. For example, facing a life-threatening situation or dealing with a family emergency can kickstart the sympathetic nervous system into the "fight-or-flight" mode.

When the sympathetic nervous system is activated, the epinephrine released from the adrenal gland prepares the nerves of our body for physical stress by increasing the heart rate, increasing the blood flow to the muscles, and decreasing the digestive and reproductive organs activities. This type of emotional stress which may lead to a physical stress was part of a day-to-day life for the hunter-gatherers in ancient times. Nowadays, it is still part of the lives of some tribes that live in tropical forests or other parts of the world in which our modern way of living has not yet penetrated.

Emotional stress can also be imaginary. In this case, the stress is not real, but it is perceived as being very real and is produced by our overactive brain. Neuroscience is making great progress in understanding what a thought is and what triggers it. We are unique individuals, with thoughts based on memories which are based on our past experiences. We are the sum of our experiences. Each of us has a unique way of thinking which makes us who we are. It is our identity. It determines the way we see the world. It determines our reality.

Thoughts are very complex. We usually start with an emotional, a physical feeling or even a smell and the thought triggered by that is moving at very high speed to a memory we have in our subconscious mind triggering another thought that is moving to another memory in our subconscious mind and so on and so forth. How many times did I find myself starting with a thought and getting a few minutes later, from thought to thought, to another one that has nothing to do with the subject that created the first one in my mind? Our mind is active 24/7 and we are continuously pulling out the thoughts we have already built in it, and we are continuously building new thoughts. Because of this, we need to control our thoughts and not let them build up into negative fictional scenarios that are not true and might never come true.

Unfortunately, our mind is used to go more towards pessimistic inner dialogue and makes us see more threats, and worries, more lack of confidence which creates self-induced, imaginary stress.

Given the absence of clinical diagnostics specifically for emotional stress, it becomes essential for individuals to develop a keen awareness of their emotional and physical states.

Short-term stress can be beneficial, helping us to stay focused in an interview or an exam, saving our lives when we must run from an imminent danger or hitting the brakes to avoid an accident, forcing us to outperform, if we are the competitive type, or to study.

When the emotional stress, real or imaginary, is short-term the sympathetic system stops being triggered as soon as the stressor disappears and leaves place to the parasympathetic nervous system which restores the body to a calm state of "rest and digest" and slows the heartbeat, stimulates the digestive system (stomach, intestines, liver) and relaxes the muscles.

If the emotional stress continues for a long period of time the body does not go into the normal, calmer state and the digestive system, amongst others, is slowed down, the contractions of its muscles and the secretions for digestion are reduced. The food goes through the esophagus into the stomach and from here into the small intestine not completely digested. We might feel our stomach is hurting or we might feel indigestion. Some of us feel heartburn and some don't. The undigested food normally causes diarrhea and abdominal cramps as well. These symptoms are not exclusive to being in a state of stress for a long period of time, they are also specific to other causes like gut flora imbalance, certain minerals or enzyme deficiencies, and some intestinal parasites. That is why it is important to find a good doctor that is a good diagnostician.

The human body is a complex and perfect mechanism. When everything is in equilibrium all our organs, hormones and body functions work in harmony. When the balance is disturbed our physical body in conjunction with our unconscious part of the brain try to rebalance the whole system compensating in one area by reducing activity in another. If this stress goes on for a longer period of time the whole balance is broken, and we start feeling its effects manifesting like physical or mental diseases.

There is no definition of what the length of a short-term stress is. Since we are so different and each of us have our own threshold, physical or emotional, the "short term" may vary from one week to several months. Our tolerance to stress is determined by our life experiences, our attitude, our perceptions. "What doesn't kill you makes you stronger" is not valid for everyone.

One alarm signal to look for is when the emotional stress changes into a physical stress. A headache, an upper back pain, diarrhea, bloating, acid reflux, heartburn, a stomach or abdominal cramp that go on for a short period of time or for several days. All these are signs that your body is for too long into a "fight or flight" state, and you have to stop, reassess your diet and lifestyle and make a change if needed. Since I loved what I did at work I did not realize the day-to-day stress piled up to the point where my health was at risk. I started to have pain behind my sternum to the point that I could not sleep. The pain was going on and off for about a week, so I did not take it seriously thinking that was only something I ate. It was though my body reacting to the stress I was unconsciously feeling.

Another alarm signal is the sleep pattern. If you normally sleep seven to eight hours every night and you start waking up during the night two to three times per week this can be another warning sign the body and mind gives you that you might be stressed.

Blood tests give as well information regarding the level of stress we are in. The DHEA/cortisol ratio is an indicator that stress affects our hypothalamic-pituitary-adrenal (HPA) axis. If stress is unmanaged and harmful, the DHEA/cortisol ratio drops and vice versa. Also, bad toxic stress increases the homocysteine and cortisol into the blood.

There is more and more evidence-based information about the mind-brain-body connection. What we think, feel, choose to say or do, directly and indirectly, affects our brain and body.

If the stress is not managed, it can create a low-grade inflammation into our bodies which increases our probability of having an autoimmune disease.

Stress not only affects our emotional state but can also lead to negative behavioral patterns, which in turn can have detrimental long-term health consequences.

When under stress, many individuals may turn to coping mechanisms like overeating, excessive drinking, or drug use as temporary escapes from their problems. While these behaviors might provide short-term relief or distraction, they can significantly exacerbate stress levels and overall health in the long run.

Overeating, especially unhealthy foods, can lead to weight gain and increase the risk of various health issues, including heart disease, high blood pressure, and type 2 diabetes. Stress eating is often a response to emotional discomfort rather than physical hunger, and it can become a harmful cycle where the stress triggers overeating, which in turn leads to more stress due to health concerns or weight gain.

Similarly, turning to alcohol or drugs as a means of coping with stress can create additional health problems. While they may seem to offer a temporary reprieve from stress, they often impair judgment, exacerbate anxiety and depression, and can lead to dependency. Excessive drinking can cause liver damage, increase the risk of certain cancers, and affect cardiovascular health. Drug abuse can have a myriad of negative effects on both physical and mental health and can lead to addiction.

It's crucial to develop positive coping mechanisms such as exercise, meditation, engaging in hobbies, or seeking support from friends, family, or professionals.

2.2.2 HOW TO MANAGE STRESS

"Wellness is really about balancing our mind, body, and spirit. It's learning about who you are and finding happiness. Wellness is charting a path towards health with a positive outlook. It's about living your life to the fullest."

Susan Blum, MD, MPH, Functional Medicine Doctor, and Founder of Blum Center for Health

Have you ever encountered a situation where you had to interact with a person who was a bully, disrespectful, and arrogant? Perhaps a 'know-it-all' type? If so, you might have experienced an accelerated heartbeat approaching the meeting room, felt blood rush to your head upon entering, and noticed your breathing become faster and shallower, especially when trying to speak. Such situations, though intense, are typically short-lived. After leaving the meeting, you might ruminate for a day or two about the exchange, but if you don't encounter that person again soon, your stress level gradually decreases, allowing your body to return to equilibrium and your breathing to become deeper and more diaphragmatic.

If you can't relate to that example, consider yourself fortunate. Maybe you've experienced the nerves of making a presentation to upper management, feeling unprepared and fearful of not performing optimally, or the anxiety of going into an exam underprepared, with your stomach in knots. These are all instances of acute, short-term stress.

In my own experience with similar stressful situations, I initially turned to breathing exercises. However, they seemed ineffective, leading me to doubt my ability to handle stress maturely. As someone who thrives on problem-solving and overcoming challenges, I attempted to reframe these stressful situations as opportunities to calm myself and achieve a relaxed state. Despite my efforts, including practices like yoga, meditation, and nature walks, I found myself increasingly stressed. The more I focused on calming down and employing breathing exercises, the more anxious I became.

Eventually, I uncovered the key reason behind the ineffectiveness of my stress management attempts: inconsistency. Just as tennis players and athletes in general need regular practice before a tournament, stress-relief techniques like breathing exercises require consistent practice to be effective. I realized that sporadic attempts at these exercises, particularly only during moments of high stress, were insufficient. The same principle applied to meditation, yoga, and walking; these activities demand a presence of mind and a disconnection from ongoing negative or stressful thoughts.

Understanding this, I began to approach these practices differently. Rather than waiting for stress to peak, I integrated them into my daily routine. Regular practice helped me not only in mastering these techniques but also in preventing the buildup of stress. By consistently engaging in these activities, I learned to be in the moment, effectively quieting my mind and reducing the impact of stress.

Here are several techniques for stress relief:

Breathing: Breathing plays a fundamental role in regulating our body's response to stress and relaxation. The process of inhalation involves expanding the lungs and pushing down the diaphragm, which can inadvertently increase the heart rate and stimulate the sympathetic nervous system. This system is often referred to as the 'fight or flight' response, preparing the body for action and alertness. However, this state is not conducive to relaxation.

To induce a state of calm, it's the parasympathetic nervous system that needs to be activated. This system is responsible for the 'rest and digest' functions of the body. One of the most effective ways to engage this system is through controlled, prolonged exhalations. When we exhale slowly and for a longer duration than our inhalation, it sends a signal to the brain that helps to relax the body and decrease the heart rate. This process can be particularly effective if accompanied by long sighs, which further enhance the relaxation response.

Mindfulness in breathing, focusing on both the inhalation and exhalation, is a simple yet powerful tool to regulate our body's stress response. The technique I follow involves a conscious effort to control the breathing pattern. I start by inhaling for a count of 4-5, ensuring that my belly expands first, which is a sign of engaging the diaphragm effectively. This type of breathing is known as diaphragmatic breathing, which is essential for deep, effective breaths. After the inhalation, I held my breath for a short count of 2-3. This pause allows for a moment of stillness and can increase the absorption of oxygen. Finally, the key part of the process is the exhalation, which I extend for a count of 6-8 or sometimes even longer. This prolonged exhalation is where the activation of the parasympathetic nervous system really comes into play, helping to bring about a sense of calm and relaxation.

This breathing technique, while simple, requires practice and mindfulness to become a natural response to stress. Regular practice can make it an automatic response to stressful situations, aiding in quicker relaxation and better management of stress. Additionally, this kind of controlled breathing has broader health benefits, such as improving lung function, reducing blood pressure, and enhancing overall emotional well-being. It is a powerful tool that we always have at our disposal, requiring no equipment or special environment to practice.

Meditation is widely recognized as a highly effective tool for reducing stress levels. Among the various forms of meditation, yoga Nidra is particularly beneficial for this purpose. This guided meditation, which I practice regularly before going to bed, involves a deep state of relaxation while maintaining consciousness. It helps in systematically calming the body and mind, leading to significant stress relief and improved mental clarity.

Another effective technique is the body scan meditation. This method focuses on progressively relaxing different parts of the body, promoting an overall sense of calm. It's particularly useful for those who experience physical manifestations of stress, as it encourages awareness and release of tension in the body. Both yoga Nidra and body scan meditations can be easily found on platforms like

YouTube, offering guided sessions suitable for both beginners and experienced practitioners.

To fully benefit from meditation, consistency is key. While longer sessions can be more immersive, shorter sessions of 5 to 10 minutes can also be quite effective, especially for those with busy schedules. These brief sessions can serve as a quick reset for the mind, helping to clear thoughts and alleviate stress. Closing your eyes, focusing on your breathing, and being mindful of your immediate surroundings during these sessions can significantly enhance their effectiveness.

The beauty of meditation lies in its diversity. There are numerous types of meditation practices, each with unique characteristics and benefits. If a particular style, like mindfulness meditation or transcendental meditation, doesn't seem to fit your needs, it's worthwhile to explore others. For instance, some people may find movement-based meditations, such as walking meditation or tai chi, more engaging.

In addition to reducing stress, regular meditation has been shown to lower blood pressure, reduce inflammation, and improve mood and sleep quality. These physical health benefits, coupled with enhanced mental clarity and emotional stability, make meditation a holistic approach to well-being.

In my own journey, incorporating meditation into my daily routine has been transformative. I've noticed a marked improvement in my ability to handle stress and my overall mental health. While initially, some practices didn't resonate with me, experimenting with different types and being patient in finding what worked best was key to my success.

Exercising and engaging in outdoor activities like walking in nature are not only beneficial for physical health but also play a significant role in enhancing mental well-being. When we exercise or take a leisurely walk amidst natural surroundings, our body releases a variety of chemicals that contribute to a sense of calm and relaxation.

One of the key chemicals released during physical activity is endorphins, often referred to as the body's natural painkillers. These chemicals interact with the receptors in the brain to reduce the perception of pain and trigger a positive feeling in the body, similar to that of morphine. This endorphin release can lead to what is commonly known as the "runner's high," a feeling of euphoria that can follow intense physical activity.

Additionally, spending time in nature, away from the hustle and bustle of daily life, can significantly reduce stress levels. Natural settings have a calming effect on the mind, helping to reduce feelings of anxiety and depression. The tranquility of nature, combined with the physical activity of walking, contributes to lowering cortisol levels, the body's primary stress hormone. This reduction in cortisol levels is crucial for achieving a state of calm and relaxation.

Being mindful of the environment while walking in nature amplifies these benefits. Mindfulness involves being fully present and engaged in the moment, aware of your surroundings and sensations without judgment. This practice can help quieten the mind, bringing attention away from stressors and redirecting it towards the beauty and serenity of the natural world.

Furthermore, exposure to sunlight during outdoor activities can boost serotonin levels, a neurotransmitter associated with boosting mood and helping a person feel calm and focused. Sunlight is also vital for vitamin D production, which plays a role in mood regulation.

Laughing indeed serves as an excellent therapy against stress, harnessing the power of humor to bring about physical and emotional relief. Laughter triggers a cascade of positive effects in the body, reinforcing the saying that 'laughter is the best medicine'.

When we laugh, our body releases endorphins, the brain's natural feel-good chemicals. These endorphins promote an overall sense of well-being and can temporarily relieve pain. Laughter also stimulates circulation and aids muscle relaxation, both of which help reduce the physical symptoms of stress.

However, initiating laughter can sometimes be challenging, especially during periods of anxiety or low mood. In such cases, simply smiling can be a powerful starting point. Smiling, even artificially, can have a surprisingly positive impact. When we smile, our brain releases dopamine and serotonin, neurotransmitters that contribute to feelings of happiness and relaxation. This act, even if it's just turning up the corners of the mouth, can kickstart the parasympathetic nervous system. This activation helps the body to slow down, counteracting the effects of the stress-induced "fight or flight" response.

Moreover, the physical act of smiling, even without genuine amusement or joy, can send a feedback signal to the brain that enhances mood. This phenomenon is known as the facial feedback hypothesis, where the brain interprets the positioning of facial muscles as an indication of emotion, and in response, can alter one's emotional state.

Incorporating laughter into daily life doesn't always require a specific reason or stimulus. Watching a funny movie, reading a humorous book, or even engaging in laughter yoga, a practice that involves prolonged voluntary laughter, can be effective ways to induce laughter and enjoy its stress-relieving benefits.

Controlling negative thoughts and behaviors is indeed a challenging but crucial aspect of managing emotional stress. Negative thoughts can create a cycle of stress and anxiety, impacting our overall well-being. To break this cycle and foster a more positive outlook, several effective techniques can be employed.

One such technique is reframing the situation. This involves consciously shifting your perspective to view challenges or stressful situations in a more positive or constructive light. For example, instead of viewing a difficult task as an insurmountable problem, you can see it as an opportunity to learn and grow. This shift in perspective can reduce feelings of stress and help you approach situations with a more positive mindset.

Surrounding yourself with positive people is another effective strategy. The company we keep can significantly influence our mood and outlook on life. Being around optimistic and supportive individuals can uplift your spirits and provide a more positive environment, which in turn can help in mitigating stress and negative thoughts.

Journaling or writing down your thoughts is a powerful tool for self-reflection and stress management. When you write down what's troubling you, it helps in organizing your thoughts and can provide clarity. Once your thoughts are on paper, challenge them by questioning their validity and looking for evidence that contradicts these negative beliefs. This practice can help in identifying and altering cognitive distortions, leading to more rational and positive thinking.

Practicing gratitude is also a profound way to shift focus from negative to positive. By taking time each day to reflect on and acknowledge the things you are thankful for, you can cultivate a sense of contentment and reduce stress. Gratitude helps in recognizing the positive aspects of life, balancing out negative thoughts and emotions.

Overall, mastering our mind and taking control over our feelings is an ongoing process that requires practice and patience. By adopting these techniques and incorporating them into daily life, you can significantly reduce emotional stress and foster a more positive, resilient mindset.

Calming music is indeed a widely recognized and effective tool for stress relief and relaxation. Different genres of music, such as jazz, classical, meditative tunes, or even personal favorites, can have a soothing impact on many individuals. The power of music to influence mood and emotional states is well-documented and can be a simple yet profound way to alleviate stress and promote calmness.

Aromatherapy, a practice dating back to ancient times, utilizes essential oils derived from plants for therapeutic purposes, including stress relief. This natural approach to wellness taps into the potent properties of plant essences to influence mood, emotional well-being, and overall health.

Popular oils for stress relief include lavender, known for its calming and soothing properties; chamomile, renowned for its relaxation and sleep-promoting effects; and peppermint, often used for its refreshing and invigorating qualities. Each oil has its own unique benefits and can be used individually or blended together for more complex aromas and effects.

However, it's important to exercise caution with aromatherapy, especially when considering air quality. Commercially available air fresheners, although convenient, often contain synthetic fragrances and chemicals that can be harmful when inhaled. These products might mask odors but do not provide the therapeutic benefits of natural essential oils. In contrast, aromatherapy using pure essential oils is a more natural and health-conscious approach to enhancing air quality and mental well-being.

Foot soak or a full body soak. A foot soak or a full body soak can indeed be a highly relaxing and rejuvenating experience, particularly after a long day of work. Incorporating Epsom salts or Magnesium chloride into these soaks enhances their calming and therapeutic effects.

Epsom salts, scientifically known as magnesium sulfate, are well-known for their relaxation properties. When dissolved in warm water, Epsom salts break down into magnesium and sulfate. Soaking in this solution allows your body to absorb the magnesium through the skin, which can help reduce muscle soreness, alleviate stress, and promote relaxation. Magnesium plays a critical role in various bodily functions, including muscle and nerve function, and is also known for its ability to improve sleep quality.

Similarly, Magnesium chloride, another form of magnesium, can also be used in soaks. Like Epsom salts, it offers the benefits of magnesium when absorbed through the skin. Magnesium chloride is often preferred by some for its higher levels of bioavailability, meaning the body may absorb it more efficiently compared to magnesium sulfate.

For a foot soak, simply fill a basin with warm water and add a cup of Epsom salts or Magnesium chloride, allowing them to dissolve completely. Submerge your feet for about 20-30 minutes, allowing yourself to relax and unwind. For a full body experience, draw a warm bath and add two cups of the salts, soaking for the same duration. This not only helps in relaxing the muscles and calming the mind but also can be beneficial for skin health.

Having a strong social support network, comprising friends and family, is a crucial method for relieving stress and enhancing overall well-being. The ability to share your worries, thoughts, and feelings with trusted individuals, without the fear of judgment, provides significant emotional relief and support.

The presence of a robust support system offers numerous benefits in managing stress. Firstly, it provides a sense of belonging and connectedness, which is fundamental to emotional health. Knowing that there are people who care and are willing to listen can make challenging situations feel more manageable.

Secondly, sharing problems or concerns with others can provide new perspectives and insights. Friends and family can offer advice, empathy, or simply a different viewpoint, which can be invaluable in seeing problems in a new light and finding solutions.

Moreover, social interactions themselves can be inherently stress-relieving. Engaging in conversations, participating in shared activities, or simply spending quality time with loved ones can elevate mood, reduce feelings of isolation, and trigger the release of endorphins, the body's natural feel-good chemicals.

Good social support also contributes to resilience, which is the ability to bounce back from stressful situations. People with strong social networks often find it easier to navigate through life's challenges and recover from setbacks thanks to the emotional and practical support they receive.

However, it's important to cultivate healthy, supportive relationships. Quality of relationships matters more than quantity. Surrounding yourself with positive, understanding, and non-judgmental people is key. This means nurturing relationships that provide mutual respect, understanding, and positivity.

Massage: Receiving a massage is a profoundly effective way to reduce stress. It can alleviate muscle tension, improve circulation, and promote relaxation. The therapeutic touch of a massage can also trigger the release of endorphins, reducing feelings of stress and anxiety.

Sauna: Spending time in a sauna is another relaxing activity. The heat of a sauna can help relax muscles, release tension, and promote sweating, which is a natural way for the body to detoxify. The warmth and quiet environment of a sauna also provides an excellent setting for relaxation and mental unwinding.

Solving Puzzles: Engaging in puzzles, such as jigsaw puzzles, crosswords, or sudoku is a great way to divert the mind from stressors. This activity requires concentration and problem-solving, providing a mental distraction and a sense of accomplishment upon completion. It can also be a meditative process, as it requires focus and patience.

Kneading Dough or Squeezing a Stress Ball: These simple physical activities can be surprisingly effective in managing stress. The repetitive motion of kneading dough or squeezing a stress ball can be a physical outlet for stress and tension. These activities can also be meditative, providing a break from intense mental focus.

Sipping Herbal Tea or a Smoothie: The act of slowly drinking a comforting beverage like herbal tea or a smoothie can be very calming. Herbal teas, such as chamomile or peppermint, are known for their natural stress-relieving properties. The ritual of preparing and enjoying a drink can also provide a much-needed pause in a busy day so long as it is done mindfully.

In our modern, fast-paced world, the ability to navigate and manage different forms of stress is crucial for maintaining overall well-being. Stress management is not just about dealing with immediate stressors but also about cultivating a lifestyle and mindset that can preemptively mitigate the onset of stress. This involves creating a balance between work, personal life, and leisure, ensuring that each area receives adequate attention and time.

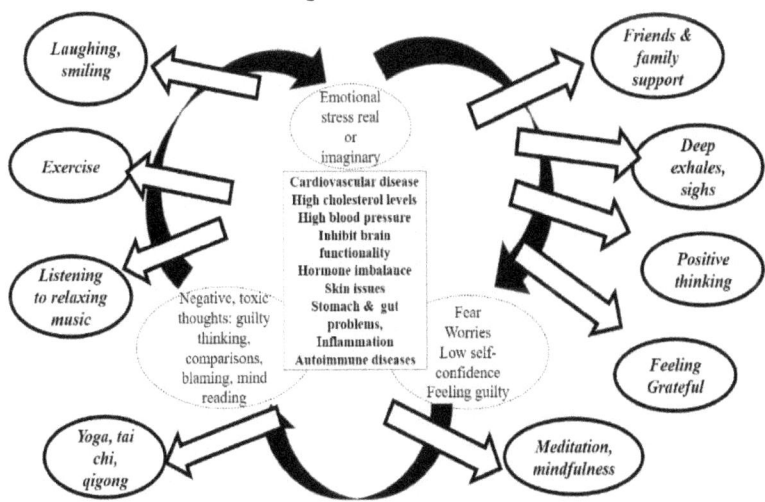

2.3 MY REAL TROUBLES ARE JUST STARTING

In engineering, failing to fix a malfunctioning system, typically the root cause, is not an option. Physicians often struggle to completely resolve their patients' health problems, frequently resorting to prescribing a mix of medications for symptom relief that, in many cases, worsen the patient's condition over time.

In 2009, during a medical examination in Mexico, an endoscopy revealed irritation in the lining of my esophagus, particularly near where it joins the stomach. This initial examination was a response to the persistent pains I had been experiencing for several years. The GI doctor decided that the treatment was to take Proton Pump Inhibitors (PPIs) indefinitely. I began a daily regimen of 40mg Nexium, and I was assured that this would allow me to live a normal life, free from the pains that had been troubling me. However, during this consultation, there was a noticeable absence of discussion regarding potential stress factors or dietary influences that might have contributed to my condition.

Seeking a more comprehensive understanding of my diagnosis, I returned to Montreal and consulted another gastroenterologist. I underwent another endoscopy and biopsy, hoping this would provide more clarity. However, the results were not as definitive as I had hoped. The pathology report stated that the findings were "not conclusive for Barrett's metaplasia," which left me in a state of uncertainty. The Montreal doctor neither confirmed nor denied the initial diagnosis of Barrett's Esophagus from Mexico. Despite the ambiguity, his recommendation was to continue with the Nexium treatment. He asserted the safety of PPIs, claiming, "there is no medicine safer than a PPI, not even The Pill."

Reflecting on my experiences and frustrations with the current medical system, I often find myself comparing it to engineering practices. In discussions with friends, I've posed a question: What would happen if engineers handled problems in the same manner as some traditional medical doctors? To elaborate, consider this analogy: Imagine your washing machine is leaking and damaging your laundry room or even the basement. You call a technician who, instead of investigating the root cause, like a punctured hose or a faulty switch, simply installs a tray under the washing machine to catch the water. This approach only addresses the symptom — the leakage — but neglects the underlying issue. In the field of engineering, such superficial solutions would be unacceptable, likely leading to job termination, as identifying and fixing the root cause is critical.

This analogy serves to highlight my concern with the medical field, where treatments often rely heavily on prescribing medication. These medications, while effective in managing symptoms, frequently come with side effects. In my case, being prescribed Nexium for Barrett's Esophagus brought temporary relief but did not address the potential underlying causes of the condition. Much like the temporary fix for the washing machine, the medication was supposed to manage the symptoms without exploring deeper issues.

In contrast to this approach, there is an argument to be made for a more holistic view of health, one that considers lifestyle changes as a primary intervention. Often, alterations in diet, exercise, stress management, and other lifestyle factors can alleviate, or even resolve, health issues. Unfortunately, the tendency to quickly resort to medication can overlook these potentially effective, more natural solutions. It's important to recognize that while medication is an essential tool in healthcare, its use as a first-line treatment should be balanced with an exploration of lifestyle modifications.

The complexity of medical practice undoubtedly surpasses that of many engineering problems. Medical issues often involve multifaceted layers of biological, psychological, and social factors. However, there is growing recognition amongst people suffering with autoimmune diseases of the need for medicine to evolve, incorporating a more comprehensive approach that not only treats symptoms with medication but also addresses lifestyle factors and underlying causes.

In early 2011, after wrapping up a two-year contract in Mexico, we moved to the USA for a new job opportunity, leaving behind our loved ones in Montreal. This transition wasn't easy, marking the start of another challenging period filled with both professional pressures and profound personal losses. Losing my mother in May 2011 and my father in March 2013 was particularly tough. As an only child very close to my parents, the grief was intense, compounded by guilt over not being there during their cancer battles. This guilt, a shadow over my heart, was slightly eased by spending precious final moments with them, thanks to my employer's flexibility.

These experiences of loss and guilt, interwoven with the challenges of adapting to a new country and job, defined a significant and emotionally complex period of my life.

In the summer of 2011, I decided to seek a third opinion from a gastroenterologist in my new city. This led to yet another endoscopy and biopsy. The results this time indicated "Reflux esophagitis, no Barrett's. Z-line mild to moderately irregular, no active ulcer or stricture," with the rest of the stomach and esophagus appearing normal. The recommended treatment was a daily dose of a proton pump inhibitor (PPI) and annual endoscopies with biopsies.

Barrett's Esophagus (BE) is a condition considered precancerous, characterized by the erosion of the esophageal lining due to acid reflux. This erosion leads to the replacement of the normal esophageal tissue with tissue more akin to that of the intestinal lining, which is more resistant to stomach acid. However, Reflux esophagitis, or GERD, is a distinct condition. Typically, lifestyle changes such as diet modification, stress management, exercise, eating smaller meals, or even taking hydrochloric acid (HCL) could potentially address GERD. Surprisingly, HCL might have been a more appropriate treatment option for me, a point I'll explain further in the next chapter. Nonetheless, my treatment plan continued to revolve around daily PPI medication.

A study I came across on PubMed.gov, published in September 2009, [31], suggested an inverse relationship between gastric pH and esophageal acid exposure. This finding implies that symptoms commonly associated with acid reflux, Barrett's Esophagus, and GERD might actually indicate a lack of stomach acid rather than an excess. Consequently, prescribing acid-reducing medication could potentially hinder healing and even be more damaging in the long term.

Reflecting on this, I often wonder whether my diagnosis was actually Barrett's Esophagus or merely esophagitis. In hindsight, I believe I should have requested a gastric pH monitoring test. At that time, I was still of the mindset that doctors knew best, and I wasn't even aware that measuring stomach pH during an endoscopy was a possibility. Today, it's not standard practice to measure stomach pH before prescribing PPI medication, and some doctors might even refuse to perform this test.

The process for diagnosing Barrett's Esophagus involves two key criteria:

- the detection of a pink lining in the esophagus during an endoscopy, which extends upwards from the gastroesophageal junction (known as the Z-line).
- the identification of intestinal-type cells within a biopsy sample taken from this lining.

To his credit, the doctor I consulted in Mexico commendably provided me with the glass slide containing the cells from my biopsy, urging me to seek further opinions from other pathology labs in Montreal.

In the diagnosis of short-segment Barrett's Esophagus, there's a notable risk of mistakenly biopsying the gastric cardia (see Fig. 1), which is part of the stomach near the Z-line. This mistake can occur due to movement during the endoscopy or because of an irregular Z-line.

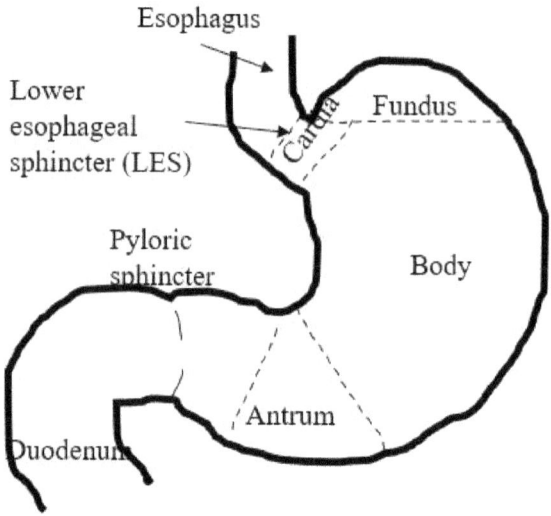

Fig. 1 Stomach areas

The cardia is the upper portion of the stomach and is composed of these columnar cells. The Z-line, which appears as a zigzag border under microscopic examination, demarcates the transition from the esophagus to the stomach. An irregular Z-line can present as columnar cells extending into the esophagus, creating a potential for misinterpretation during a biopsy. If a biopsy is erroneously taken from this area of intermixed cells, it might lead to a misdiagnosis, mistaking gastric cardia cells for Barrett's Esophagus cells.

In my case, this possibility leaves me questioning the accuracy of my diagnosis. Was my condition a case of misdiagnosed Barrett's Esophagus, or was it accurately identified? This uncertainty remains, but what is certain is that in the years that followed, I experienced numerous health issues that seemed to be misdiagnosed or not fully understood.

2.4 IT GETS WORSE BEFORE IT GETS BETTER

"Everyone has a doctor in him or her; we just have to help it in its work. The natural healing force within each one of us is the greatest force in getting well."

Hippocrates, the father of Western medicine.

From 2009 to 2013, I faithfully followed my prescribed regimen of taking Nexium, 40 mg daily, complemented by annual endoscopies. Despite this adherence, I continued to experience episodes of upper stomach pain several times a year. With each yearly endoscopy, I voiced my concerns about the long-term use of Nexium. Yet, my gastroenterologist consistently reassured me, citing the prevalence of prolonged PPI usage without adverse effects among many patients.

However, in 2013, after four years of PPI treatment, my health took a turn. I began to suffer from debilitating symptoms: overwhelming fatigue, back and abdominal pain, blurred vision, and frequent headaches. A visit to my general practitioner and subsequent blood tests uncovered a vitamin B12 deficiency. This led to a new treatment of monthly B12 injections. Notably, vitamin B12 deficiency can be a side effect of prolonged PPI use, as these medications reduce stomach acid necessary for B12 absorption. However, this potential link was not considered by any of my healthcare providers.

For a trained physician I assume it should be logical to connect the long-term use of PPIs with the impediment of vitamin and mineral absorption, including B12. Yet, this correlation was overlooked. This oversight could be attributed to the conventional medical practice's tendency to focus on specific symptoms or organs rather than adopting a holistic approach. In my experience, this meant that the interconnectedness of my symptoms and medication usage was not fully considered.

Vitamin B12 deficiency can arise from a variety of sources, including:

- Pernicious anemia, a condition where the body's immune system erroneously targets and destroys stomach parietal cells. These cells are crucial for producing intrinsic factor, a substance vital for B12 absorption in the gut.

- Imbalance in the intestinal microbiota, leading to malabsorption of B12 in the small intestine.

- Diets lacking in sufficient vitamin B12, which is predominantly found in animal products, especially liver.

- Certain medications that interfere with the secretion of intrinsic factor, hindering the absorption of vitamin B12 into the bloodstream. Without intrinsic factor, vitamin B12 cannot be efficiently transported to cells and is instead expelled from the body.

In my case, dietary deficiency was an unlikely cause. My diet has consistently been rich in vitamin B12 sources, such as meat and beef liver. Additionally, there is no known history of autoimmune diseases like pernicious anemia in my family. It's essential to note that pernicious anemia is more than a symptom of B12 deficiency; it's an autoimmune condition that actively contributes to the deficiency by impeding the body's ability to absorb the vitamin. The only logical explanation left is the medication that interferes with the secretion of intrinsic factor or/and the imbalance in the intestinal microbiota.

The use of Proton Pump Inhibitor (PPI) medication, designed to substantially reduce stomach acid by acting on the parietal cells, can significantly alter the digestion process. By reducing stomach acid by up to 95% [32], PPIs can disrupt the natural balance of bacteria in the intestinal microbiome, a condition known as dysbiosis. This imbalance can weaken the immune system, potentially increasing susceptibility to infections. Over time, such a weakened immune response could, in theory, contribute to the development of autoimmune diseases [33]. Moreover, the dysbiosis potentially induced by PPI use may have broader implications for the immune system. The imbalance in the gut microbiota can weaken the body's defenses, leading to a higher likelihood of infections. These recurring infections could, in some scenarios, trigger or exacerbate autoimmune responses.

The long-term use of PPI medication that I have been exposed to might have led to malabsorption of vitamin B12. Stomach acid plays a critical role in extracting B12 from the food we consume. Due to the acid-suppressing action of PPIs, this crucial step in vitamin B12 release into the blood may be hindered. For B12 to be absorbed into the bloodstream and then transported to cells, it must bind with the intrinsic factor. PPI can interfere with this process.

This understanding of the possible side effects of PPIs, including vitamin B12 malabsorption and its impact on the immune system, aligns with the abdominal pain, fatigue, brain fog, and blurred vision symptoms I experienced. It raises the question of whether the long-term use of PPIs was a contributing factor to my health issues and potentially to the development of an autoimmune condition. In my mind there is no doubt that the long-term use of PPIs is the main contributor to my health decline.

Vitamin B12 deficiency can lead to a range of serious health issues, such as:

- physical symptoms like tiredness, weakness, nausea, vomiting, a sore mouth, and yellowish skin.
- Neurologically, it can cause vision problems, confusion, difficulty concentrating, walking, or speaking.
- Psychologically, it may manifest as depression or irritability and, in severe cases, can be life-threatening.

While B12 injections help replenish the vitamin levels in the blood, they do not address the underlying cause of the deficiency. Treating only the symptom means the root issue remains unresolved, potentially leading to further health deterioration and progression of the disease.

As an engineer, I naturally aim to get to the bottom of issues, which led me to investigate my abdominal and back pain. Initially, I considered my history of kidney stones and consulted with a gynecologist and a urologist, but these were quickly ruled out. So, I turned my focus to my gastrointestinal (GI) tract and met with a GI specialist. During this visit, I also shared the stress I was under from my father's recent passing. The diagnosis was twofold: Barrett's Esophagus and Irritable Bowel Syndrome (IBS), the latter based purely on my symptoms, without any additional testing. The recommended treatment included Hyoscyamine sulfate, alongside my ongoing Nexium and new B12 shots. Concerned about Hyoscyamine's side effects, I chose not to take it. Three years later, feeling the need for a fresh perspective, I decided to change my GI specialist and requested my medical records for the transition. Upon reviewing them, I noticed the notes from my visit on 12/12/2013, which stated:

> *"Reviewd IBS etc with pt including antispasmodics and SSRI pt has in past been very obstinant wrt meds and staying on anything even her PPI when she stays very concerned about her Barretts."*

(Here, 'pt' refers to 'patient,' and 'wrt' to 'with regards to,' for clarification).

Before proceeding further, let's take a moment to delve into what irritable bowel syndrome (IBS) is and explore its causes.

Around 5-10% of the world's population and between 25 and 45 million people in the United States are diagnosed with IBS [34]. Irritable Bowel Syndrome (IBS) is a gastrointestinal disorder characterized by a group of symptoms that can include abdominal pain, bloating, and changes in bowel habits such as diarrhea, constipation, or alternating between the two. IBS has historically been a diagnosis of exclusion meaning that other diseases have to be ruled out in order to get an IBS diagnosis. In other words, if the doctors can't find out what is wrong with you, IBS it is. Diagnosis is based on symptoms, but these symptoms are nonspecific meaning we can see them across different conditions and diseases.

The exact cause of IBS is not well understood, but it is believed to involve a variety of factors including:

- Gut bacteria overgrowth or lack of bacteria variety.
- Intestinal muscle contractions.
- Gastrointestinal infection.
- Genetics.
- Communication between the gut and the brain.

Treatment for IBS, in theory, should involve a combination of dietary changes, lifestyle modifications, and stress management. In most cases though, medications are prescribed to relieve symptoms.

Considering my ongoing concerns about the side effects of long-term use of Proton Pump Inhibitors (PPIs) and my symptoms of abdominal pain, my doctor opted for what he thought best: prescribing medication, following the "a pill for every ill" approach. While it's true that some IBS causes, like genetics, are challenging to address naturally, other factors such as gut bacteria imbalance or gastrointestinal infections could potentially be managed with lifestyle changes, including diet modifications, probiotics, and stress control. Moreover, after years of annual endoscopies with no indication of Barrett's Esophagus, a reevaluation of my treatment seemed prudent. In hindsight, stopping the PPIs and altering my lifestyle to bring my stomach acid levels closer to normal might have been a more appropriate approach in my case. Such a strategy could have addressed the root causes of my gut problems rather than just mitigating the symptoms.

In 2016, I experienced another frustrating misdiagnosis, involving my gastroenterologist (GI), an ear, nose, and throat specialist (ENT), and my general practitioner (GP). This reflected a broader issue in U.S. healthcare, where specialists often focus too narrowly on their fields, missing the bigger picture of a patient's overall health. My GI, despite knowing about my vitamin B12 deficiency, kept prescribing strong antacids and didn't consider that my prolonged use of proton pump inhibitors (PPIs) could be causing low stomach acid, which in turn might be upsetting my gut balance. This oversight suggested a lack of holistic care, something a comprehensive stool test might have clarified but was never conducted.

When I questioned my treatment, I was quickly dismissed as depressed—a common refrain, it seems, when patients challenge traditional GI diagnoses and treatments. From 2013 to 2015, despite sticking to my prescribed PPI regimen and undergoing annual endoscopies, my symptoms worsened. By April 2014, my diagnoses included Barrett's Esophagus, unspecified Colitis, IBS, and Proctitis, yet tests like colonoscopies came back normal, and my medication remained unchanged. Fortunately, my doctor did not press me to take antidepressants, as there was "no evidence of depression, anxiety or agitation."

Dissatisfied and suspecting that my doctors were missing something crucial regarding my gastrointestinal health, I sought a second opinion from another GI doctor at the end of 2015. This new specialist recommended I stop taking PPIs, offering a divergent viewpoint from my long-standing treatment plan. After over seven years on PPIs, with my health only declining, I decided to follow this new advice. Heading into 2016, I was determined to quit all medications, hoping to see an improvement in my vitamin levels and overall health.

Ceasing Proton Pump Inhibitor (PPI) medication is a challenging process. When I decided to discontinue PPIs, I wasn't aware, nor were the doctors I consulted for a second and later on for a third opinion, of the withdrawal symptoms. These included acute stomach pain caused by the stomach secreting an excess amount of acid. I will delve deeper into the safe discontinuation of PPIs in the following chapter.

My health journey took a challenging detour when, after weaning off PPIs, I was struck down by a severe flu, leaving me bedridden with a high fever. During this illness, I fainted, and in the fall I hit my head against a wall and I woke up face down on the floor. Once the fever subsided, I was left with persistent left throat and ear pain, prompting a visit to an ENT specialist. Despite thorough examinations yielding no significant findings, I was diagnosed with Laryngopharyngeal Reflux (LPR) based on symptoms and referred back to my GI doctor.

A second ENT opinion, however, suggested that my symptoms were not due to LPR but were more likely from a Temporomandibular Joint (TMJ) disorder caused by the impact on my head and neck to the wall and floor during my fall. This expert was skeptical of the LPR diagnosis, noting the absence of typical signs of throat irritation and the localized nature of my pain.

Given my history of Barrett's Esophagus and recent cessation of PPIs, I was torn about dismissing the GI angle entirely. Despite doubts about my long-standing GI doctor's approach, I decided to consult him again, driven by caution and my extensive medical history with him. In May 2016, I shared my experiences and the advice from the other GI doctor to stop PPIs, only to be met with a decision to double my PPI dosage to 40 mg twice daily. My attempt to provide a full picture of my health developments, including the fall, was dismissed, and my doctor seemed to ignore the possibility that my symptoms could be related to the physical injury rather than acid reflux. This response, along with the disregard for potential consequences of long-term acid blocker use, added to my frustration and doubts about the treatment direction.

His notes reflected irritation at being questioned:

> *"Wanted to review all of the past and even went to October of 2015. Weaned off Nexium because he found nothing!! Now off Nexium completely for 3 months. Had a flu this year as well as fell and fractured her 2 front teeth. W/U for thyroid. Also saw ENT w DL and CT."*

A few weeks later, still on the maximum PPI dose with no relief, I felt stuck and uncertain about my diagnosis. Then, during a casual visit with a friend, I met a doctor who offered a fresh perspective. He listened carefully to my story, asked pointed questions, and suggested a deeper discussion at his office.

In our meeting, he delved into the specifics of my condition, questioning the unilateral nature of my throat and ear pain and doubting the Laryngopharyngeal Reflux (LPR) diagnosis since the

ENT exam found nothing unusual. Considering my high PPI dosage, he was puzzled why my gastrin levels, which could indicate excessive acid production, hadn't been checked. He also noted the absence of any investigations into stomach emptying issues or gallbladder problems and pointed out the long-term PPI use risks like anemias, low magnesium, and bone density loss, none of which had been fully explored.

He hadn't seen any attempts to check for anatomical issues through an esophagram or upper GI X-rays. His advice was to see a headache neurologist, suspecting my symptoms might be from Glossopharyngeal neuralgia, possibly triggered by my fall. This condition, involving nerve pain in the throat and ear, matched the intermittent but intense pain I experienced, which I found bearable without medication due to potential side effects of painkillers.

This new perspective from the doctor was a stark contrast to my previous medical experiences. Unlike other consultations where LPR was hastily concluded, he took a more investigative approach. I realized again how the discrepancy between diagnoses highlights the complexities of medical evaluations, the importance of having good investigative-approach doctors and, the importance for the doctors to listen to the patient's experience and take it seriously before giving a diagnosis.

It was clear that returning to the GI doctor I had been consulting for the past six years was no longer an option for me. I had lost faith in his approach. He seemed to lack the ability to view me as a whole, as an individual with unique health needs, and appeared either unwilling or unable to identify the underlying causes of my health issues. His default response seemed to be prescribing medication for everything – the most potent acid suppressors (PPIs) and antidepressants (SSRIs). Despite this medication regimen since 2009, my abdominal discomfort not only persisted but it got worse. I continued to experience the same upper abdominal pain several times a year, and since 2013, new symptoms emerged that I hadn't dealt with before: bloating, a persistent feeling of fullness after meals, and abdominal pain.

In my quest for clarity amid conflicting medical opinions on the need for PPI medication and the reality of my Barrett's Esophagus diagnosis, I sought out a third GI specialist in September 2016. The consultation led to another endoscopy, after which the new GI doctor recommended discontinuing the PPIs, mirroring the advice of one of the previous doctors and bringing a semblance of consensus. Despite my concerns about the long-term use of PPIs, this endoscopy did reveal gastric polyps and erythematous mucosa in my stomach's antrum. This third GI specialist became my go-to for the next six years.

A year later, a follow-up endoscopy showed no evidence of Barrett's Esophagus, altering my healthcare strategy towards less invasive monitoring. For the first time since 2009, I was told I didn't have Barrett's and learned that yearly endoscopies weren't necessary, saving me from their cost and risks like infection and potential perforations.

However, neither this doctor nor the second-opinion specialist advised on how to safely quit PPIs. I learned the hard way about the harsh rebound effect of stopping them abruptly, which caused severe acid indigestion. I'll share how I managed to carefully wean off the medication in the next part of my story, navigating through the complexities of treatment cessation.

The lack of stomach acid crates a waterfall of health issues: vitamin and mineral deficiencies, poor nutrition absorption, gut microbiome imbalances, relative intestinal permeability also known as leaky gut, gallbladder and pancreas malfunction, fatty liver, stomach cancer and can lead to the development of autoimmune diseases.

The body is complex and interconnected and the gastrointestinal system sits at the core of it all.

It is connected to everything and influences functions in your body from metabolism and gut immunity to cardiovascular, skin, respiratory and urogenital health and even the brain.

Unfortunately, I did not have the curiosity to study more on this subject until 2020 when my health deteriorated too much.

In 2016, after seven years of PPI medication, my body was deprived of nutrients, the gut bacteria were altered, the intestinal wall barrier was breached, and it triggered an immune response and inflammation. This inflammation combined with the flu generated an autoimmune response that attacked not only the flu virus but also my thyroid.

Until 2016 I had only one vitamin deficiency: B12. Nobody explained to me what such a deficiency means or why I got it other than if I take B12 vitamin everything is solved. By stopping the PPI I thought this deficiency would be solved without the need for vitamin supplement. Unfortunately, it was too late for my body to recover after so many years of medication abuse.

After the fever went away, towards the end of 2016 I started to feel very, very tired, and weak. I started to lose my hair, I could not concentrate, my muscles were sore, I could not speak, I could barely walk from one room to another, I had difficulties breathing. Worried, I scheduled an appointment with my GP who ordered some blood tests. I was at work and will never forget the moment I received his phone call and announced that I had Hashimoto's, but I should not be worried because it is treatable, so he sent me to see an endocrinologist.

Believing that a university professor would be more aware of the recent advancements in his field, I sought help from a friend to arrange an appointment for me. The endocrinologist, who was also a professor at one of the local big universities, reviewed my latest blood test results and noted that my thyroid antibodies, at a level of 197, were not high enough to warrant medication. 'There are people with TPO levels over 1000. You'll need medication, but not right now,' he said. However, he didn't offer any advice regarding diet or lifestyle changes. Consequently, I left feeling just as miserable as before, plagued by weakness, dizziness, and an overwhelming lack of energy that made even speaking a challenge.

Weeks later, after time lost in another doctor's appointments and money spent on blood tests, I have been prescribed Synthroid, a medication that I have to take for life to replace a hormone that is made by the thyroid gland.

The endocrinologist, like his GP, GI and ENT colleagues, treated the symptom of the Hashimoto disease and not the cause so, he jumped to prescribe medication.

To treat Hashimoto, as well as any autoimmune disease we need to calm down the inflammation in our body first. Without quenching the inflammation, the immune system will continue attacking different parts of our body and we will end with a debilitating plethora of autoimmune diseases which will cut our lives short.

So now, I have an officially diagnosed autoimmune disease: Hashimoto. I had medication for it, but I did not have any root cause identified!

As I mentioned earlier, in late 2016, I embarked on my second attempt to gradually wean off PPIs, but the journey was more difficult and painful. My doctors' advice was simply to stop the medication, which I followed. However, a week after completely stopping the PPIs, I experienced intense stomach pain, a common result of acid rebound hypersecretion, which often correlates with the degree of prior acid inhibition.

Realizing I needed a structured plan to safely transition off acid suppressants, I logically devised a schedule to reduce PPI usage and gradually introduce H2-blocker medication (Ranitidine, Famotidine). It took more than six months now, but eventually, I was free from PPIs. Still, cautious about completely stopping acid suppression, I continued with the H2-blockers until my scheduled endoscopy in 2019.

While this self-managed approach eventually worked for me, it's crucial to emphasize the importance of medical supervision when altering such medications. Abrupt changes can have significant health implications, and while H2-blockers are generally seen as having fewer long-term side effects than PPIs, they are still potent medications that require careful handling. The endoscopy in 2019 was intended to assess the impact of these changes on my gastrointestinal health, closing one chapter of my medication journey and ensuring my approach was aligned with my current health status.

I felt it was crucial to share my experiences with misdiagnoses, prescribed medications, and their adverse effects to highlight the significance of listening to patients, considering their overall health, and applying logical reasoning in formulating a diagnosis and treatment plan.

2.5 PRESCRIPTION MEDICATION AS A TRIGGER FOR HEALTH ISSUES

Doctors hold a significant responsibility in prescribing powerful prescription medications. While often beneficial, there is no medication without serious side effects that sometimes can lead to health complications and even death.

As far as I know, there is no medication without having some harmful effects on our health. All prescription medications, supplements or even natural remedies have side effects that we will discover sooner or later in the form of unwanted symptoms and damaged health. In addition to the side effects triggered by a medication itself, the interaction between all the medicine a person takes can bring further health problems.

Many people think they are safe if they replace the medication with supplements since they come from natural sources.

This is false!

Most of the supplements are made of botanical plants and I agree they are more natural and safer than the man-made synthetic chemicals. However, even plants give us side effects if we don't take them properly or if we have other health conditions. Take Ashwagandha for example. It is a shrub that grows in Africa and Asia and is often recommended by functional dietitians for many conditions related to stress, anxiety, and insomnia. Even if it has some benefits, it does also have side effects if it is taken in large quantities like stomach upset, diarrhea, vomiting or even liver problems. It can also cause the autoimmune system to become more active therefore it is unsafe to use it if you have an autoimmune disease or if you are pregnant.

Supplements interact as well with certain medications. For example, some antioxidant supplements (vitamins C and E) might reduce the effect of some chemotherapy treatments, also vitamin A if taken in large doses can be harmful. Therefore, it's crucial to approach all medical treatments, including natural supplements, with awareness and caution, understanding their potential impact on our health.

I want to be clear on something! I do not promote stopping the medication if you already take any, but I do strongly suggest informing yourself and seeking other opinions, most importantly seek the opinion of a functional/integral medicine doctor. You might be surprised, as I was, at the benefits of switching from a hard-chemical prescription to a more soft-natural supplement. The only downsize with the supplements is that they require a special diet and life habit changes to work, and it takes longer to see the benefits than if you take a man-made-chemical pill. When I did not have any hope from the traditional medicine to understand WHY my body wanted so much to hurt itself and all I got from my traditional doctors was the same medication that brought me to where I was, I reluctantly sought the opinion of a functional/integrative doctor MD. The results were AMAZING: six months later I was cured of some abdominal pains, I did not experience any more fatigue, brain fog, I was able to play tennis one to two hours a day, three-four times per week, and, 12 months later my thyroid antibodies were going down and I was feeling GREAT and most importantly, HOPEFUL!

2.5.1 WHY MAN-MADE CHEMICAL MEDICATION IS NOT GOOD

Today's healthcare system, heavily influenced by corporate interests, often sees patients caught in a cycle of numerous strong medications. This approach can sometimes lead to worsening health outcomes, including death.

I want to reiterate a point I've made previously: every synthetic medication comes with side effects, and this reality stems from several reasons.

Firstly, our understanding of the human body, though significantly advanced from the days of leech therapy, is still incomplete. We haven't fully grasped why autoimmune diseases occur or why diets high in sugar and carbohydrates impact blood cholesterol levels more than high cholesterol diets do. Consequently, many medications developed and promoted by pharmaceutical companies, and prescribed by well-intentioned traditional doctors, tend to focus on symptom relief rather than addressing the underlying causes of health issues. This approach can lead to a cascade effect, where treating one problem may inadvertently neglect or exacerbate others.

Another factor is the intricate relationship between the medical field and broader political and economic interests. The influence of pharmaceutical company lobbying is substantial, affecting public trust, as seen in the skepticism towards vaccines during the Covid-19 pandemic. Moreover, the food industry's promotion of certain dietary trends, like low-fat diets versus higher-fat, higher-protein diets, often intertwines more with economic interests than with public health concerns. This relationship of medicine, politics, and economics involves vast sums of money and complex political agendas, which can sometimes overshadow the primary goal of enhancing public health.

One example is the cholesterol-reducer statins. Even though they are effective in lowering cholesterol they have a plethora of side effects like muscle pain, digestive problems, memory loss, fatigue and so on. The tragic part is that even now the doctors are still recommending statins for people who have high cholesterol level in order to reduce their risk of a heart attack or stroke despite the fact that there are studies showing that "lowering cholesterol has a very limited benefit in populations other than middle-aged men with a history of heart disease" [36].

Another example of medication that has a lot of front stage lately is the acid-neutralizers and acid-suppressors. Antacids are a type of medication that neutralizes or reduces the amount of acid the stomach is producing. There are three types of antacid drugs:

- *Antacids.* They neutralize the acid in the stomach. They act fast and give short-term relief. Examples are Tums, Pepto-Bismol, Gaviscon, Rolaids.

- *H2 blockers.* They suppress the amount of acid the stomach produces in 24 hours by about 70% [37]. This drug was developed in the early 1990s by Sir James Black who received the Nobel Prize for his work. The H2-blockers act by binding to the H2 receptors found in the parietal cells interfering thus with the stimulation of the parietal cells to secrete acid by the histamine. The Examples are cimetidine, ranitidine, famotidine and nizatidine. Side effects cited in a National Library of Medicine paper [37] are mentioned as uncommon, "usually minor and include diarrhea, constipation, fatigue, drowsiness, headache and muscle aches", also some "rare cases of clinically apparent, acute liver injury". I would caution in using them for the long term.

- *Proton Pump Inhibitors (PPIs).* They suppress the amount of acid the stomach produces in 24 hours by up to 95%. The parietal cells found in the fundus of our stomach produce and secrete hydrochloric acid (HCL) through a mechanism known as proton pump. The PPIs block the acid secretion action of the proton pump mechanism, thereby increasing the stomach pH (more on this in the next section of this book). **Examples of PPIs:** Omeprazole (Prilosec),

Esomeprazole (Nexium), Lansoprazole (Prevacid), Dexlansoprazole (Dexilant), Pantoprazole (Protonix), Esomeprazole (Vimovo). The side effects described in a MedlinePlus article on PPIs are "rare", headache, diarrhea, constipation, nausea, or itching [38]. Ask your provider about possible concerns with long-term use, such as infections and bone fractures". An article published and updated on April 15, 2019, in National Library of Medicine [32] mentions that "Oral forms of the PPIs are rapidly absorbed and decrease gastric acidity by 80% to 95%, although peak inhibition may require several days". It continues specifying the PPIs are "extremely well tolerated and associated with few adverse effects". I would strongly caution in using this type of medication unless you really need it and even then, not for more than a very limited amount of time (14 days). There is a lot of information about the life-threatening side effects of long-term use of PPIs. I was kept on PPIs by my doctor for seven years, believe me when I say I am one of the living proofs of the side effects of PPIs. Thanks to my healthy body and to my inquiring nature to understand the root cause of my symptoms I am still alive today.

The H2 blockers and PPIs are the medicine that traditional doctors prescribe as a first line of defense for the treatment of:

- Gastroesophageal reflux disease (GERD)
- Esophagitis produced by acid reflux
- Duodenal and gastric ulcer
- Gastritis
- Helicobacter pylori (H.pylori) eradication to reduce the risk of duodenal ulcer due to antibiotics.

Some of the above acid-suppressing medicines are available over the counter which makes it easy for normal people to auto-medicate if they feel an uncomfortable symptom after a meal. The pharmaceutical industry is paying hundreds of millions of dollars each year on research and advertising acid reducing medication. We are used to seeing on TV commercials that are pushing acid suppressor to the public: taking only one Nexium pill we'll get rid of any heartburn for 24 hours, Zantac 360 is taking away your heartburn within 15 minutes, Prilosec OTC blocks the heartburn all day.

What great options we have! We can eat everything we want, and our pain goes away with only one pill.

Proton Pump Inhibitors (PPIs) represent a significant segment of the pharmaceutical market in the United States, potentially amounting to billions of dollars annually. These medications are widely used, with a substantial portion of the population, possibly exceeding 5%, using them either through prescriptions or as over-the-counter purchases.

For some acute conditions the use of acid-suppressing medication can be useful but only if it is taken for a short period of time. The FDA recommendation is to take Nexium for 14 days at a time and "not for more than three 14-day courses in a year". This is like playing yo-yo with the acid in your stomach, disrupting the natural stomach and intestines environment and leading to maldigestion, malabsorption and malnutrition.

In case of a chronic condition when acid-suppressing medication is prescribed to be taken long-term I suggest challenging your doctor and being your own advocate to understand what the root cause of your health condition is. Always ask "what is the root cause of this bad test result". Long-term use of PPIs can cause serious health complications like vitamin and mineral deficiencies such as vitamins B12, calcium, iron and magnesium, SIBO (Small Intestinal Bacterial Overgrowth) which can lead to gastrointestinal infections, kidneys failures, osteoporosis, Hashimoto's and other autoimmune diseases.

The irony is that approximately 90% of the patients with GERD that are prescribed PPIs suffer from low stomach acid and not too much stomach acid levels as it is commonly believed, according to Dr. Jonathan Wright [39]. By prescribing PPIs to these people who have already low stomach acid they will have further acid reduction which is sending them directly into the desperation of health complications.

This makes no sense!

The biggest problem with acid-suppressing medication is that they are prescribed without any tests to evaluate if the acid reflux or indigestion is caused by low or high stomach acid production. I consulted five GI doctors and none of them did any test to measure my stomach ph. However, five out of five prescribed me PPIs to take for life.

Interesting to mention also that the acid secretion diminishes with age so much that by the time we are in our 50s, the stomach acid secretion is down by almost half compared to when we are in our 20s. Add to this an H-2 blocker or a PPI prescription and the risk of severe chronic diseases is guaranteed.

2.5.2 STRATEGY TO STOP TAKING PPIs

Many illnesses that could potentially be prevented are often managed through a system heavily reliant on prescription medications, leading to significant profits in the pharmaceutical industry.

Before you stop taking PPIs you must consult with your doctor and be your own advocate. Your need to understand why the doctor is prescribing you this type of medication and you can ask him/her the following questions:

1. What are the tests the doctor performed on you?

2. Do those results show the root cause of the health issue you are facing now or only the symptom? For example, a B12 deficiency in the blood test shows only that your body does not assimilate vitamin B12, but it does not show the real cause of this deficiency, why the B12 is not assimilated? Another example is abdominal pain that most often the GI doctors are parking it in the IBS diagnostic. Did the doctor do any stool test to understand if you have a parasite or if your microbiome is well balanced?

3. Know your body! If your instinct tells you something is not right, don't hesitate to seek a second, a third, or even a fourth opinion. You can also search on the internet what could cause certain symptoms that you are experiencing now. A good wealth of information are Facebook groups. I learned a lot from Kidney Stones, Hashimoto's, Autoimmune Gastritis and Pernicious Anemia groups. These gave me the answers I needed about my diagnostics so that I can start reading more books about them and know what to ask my doctors and how to be my own advocate. However, always critically evaluate this information and use it to complement, not replace, professional medical advice and to advocate for yourself when you feel something is off.

4. Diagnosing health issues is complex. Symptoms can overlap across different conditions, requiring doctors to be thorough and logical in their approach to detect which is the real source of your symptoms. To do this though, the doctor needs to listen to your problems since many of the symptoms can be solved without medication. I have heard a lot of people who have IBS or B12 deficiency symptoms like abdominal pain, feeling bloated, weakness, brain fog, being told by their doctors that they are depressed and prescribed antidepressants. If you feel the doctor does not listen to you don't hesitate to change him/her. Listen to your instincts!

5. Can you solve the health issue for which the doctor prescribed these acid blocker pills by changing your lifestyle and diet? Most of us prefer a quick fix solution and we are happy when the doctors give us pills. Unfortunately, we spend a lot of time living an unhealthy life (sedentary, stressful, eating badly) so it is logical that our body needs a long change to a healthy life to repair itself. We take care of the people or pets we love but we don't think about the body we live in. We inherit bad habits from the moment we are born, first directly from our family (exercise, compulsive eating, poor food choices, low stress thresholds) and then from colleagues and friends (drinking, smoking, drugs). The food we find in stores and in restaurants does not help us either. Generally, we are resistant to changes until we realize there is no other choice if we want to keep living, then we are willing to do anything, but it might be too late. The smart thing is to start living a healthy life when we are healthy. Keep in mind also that some conditions do require medication and cannot be managed by lifestyle changes alone so educate yourself.

6. Can you solve your health issue by taking less harmful medication? H2-blocker is still a dangerous anti acid medication if taken long term and I suggest not to use it for occasional heartburn after you eat a hamburger or eat at a restaurant. Tums, or magnesium carbonate or baking soda in a little water, or even a few sips of alkaline water can help with the occasional discomfort.

7. Don't hesitate to communicate openly with your doctor about your concerns regarding the diagnosis and/or the medication. According to a 2014 report from the journal BMJ Quality & Safety [35], 1 in 20 US adults are affected by diagnostic errors: "Combining estimates from the three studies yielded a rate of outpatient diagnostic errors of 5.08%, or approximately 12 million US adults every year. Based upon previous work, we estimate that about half of these errors could potentially be harmful."

Taking PPIs for an extended period, like I did for seven years, can make discontinuing them quite challenging, often resulting in severe stomach discomfort due to excess acid. When consulting doctors, I was surprised that two gastroenterologists advised me to stop taking them abruptly, or "cold turkey." This advice left me perplexed, especially considering their specialization; it was disheartening to witness a lack of detailed knowledge and apparent disinterest in the matter.

Stopping PPIs can be very difficult due to the hypersecretion of the stomach acid caused by the rebound effect. While the PPIs prevent parietal cells from secreting acid, your stomach continues to release gastrin which, if in excess leads to hyperplasia, an increase in size of the enterochromaffin-like cells (ECL). When stimulated by gastrin, the ECL cells secrete histamine in excess which in turn stimulates even more the parietal cells to produce stomach acid (HCL). Stimulated continuously by histamine, the parietal cells expand in size and have more proton pumps which means more acid secretion (more about how the stomach produces acid in the next section). Therefore, it is important not to suddenly stop the PPIs but to do it gradually.

Some people have less trouble than others to phase off PPIs. This is dependent on how long you took the acid-suppressing medication, on your own body and on your pain-standing threshold. For me it was not an easy task. When I first stopped taking the PPIs was in 2016 and I did it at the beginning, as instructed, cold turkey. I was happy to see that I had no adverse symptoms for the first week, until a couple of days later it started as a dreadful pain in my whole stomach, something I never felt before. I realized that this is the effect of the sudden stop of the medication. I restarted taking the PPI pills for few weeks, calmed my stomach by reducing again the acid in my stomach by more than 90% and, thinking in terms of a project that needed a solution, so I started making a plan:

- *Reduce the dose gradually.* I marked down on a calendar the quantity I was taking and tried to keep a certain dose for about four to five weeks so that my stomach gets used to the reduced amount. At the time I was taking 40 mg of Nexium, so I started by splitting the quantity in two-20 mg twice a day. After a month I reduced this to a single dose of 20 mg per day for another month, being very mindful of any feeling in my stomach or esophagus. From here I divided the dose into two-10 mg taken twice a day and so on and so forth. It took me close to half a year to be completely PPI-free but I was still feeling some stomach discomfort therefore my new GI doctor prescribed H2-blocker famotidine, 20 mg every morning which I took until October 2020 when I discovered the damages that the PPI and the H2-blockers did to my health (this story to continue in the next section). Replacing the PPIs with the H2-blockers can be a better choice but should be done only for a short period of time and once you feel your symptoms are under control you should gradually stop the H2-blockers as well. Below is an example of my schedule for stopping the PPI:

Week	1 to 4	5 to 8	9 to 12	13 to 16	17 to 20
Morning	40mg PPI	20mg PPI	20mg PPI	10mg PPI	20mg H2B
Evening		20mg PPI	20mg H2B	20mg H2B	20mg H2B

- During all this time I was continuously monitoring for any discomfort or reflux symptoms. I stayed vigilant for the body's response, and I observed for acid reflux. If you reduced the dose but you don't feel comfortable you can go back to the previous dose for 3-4 weeks, giving your body time to adjust, after which you can continue reducing the dose according to the schedule.

If you want to stop taking PPIs:

- Always consult with a healthcare provider before starting this schedule.
- Adjust the schedule based on individual responses and doctor's advice.
- Be mindful of potential rebound acid production and other withdrawal symptoms.
- Consider incorporating lifestyle changes, dietary adjustments, and alternative therapies to manage symptoms.

This table serves as a guideline and should be tailored to individual needs and medical advice. Regular check-ins with a healthcare provider are crucial for safely managing the process.

You can also use complementary acid-reducer options like:

1. *DGL* – Deglycyrrhizinated licorice (DGL) is a synthetic derivative of the licorice root herb, without the side effects of it: high blood pressure, potassium loss, heart problems. By removing the glycyrrhizin from the licorice root, we obtain the DGL product that has the healing properties of the plant but without its side effects. DGL has the ability to increase the secretion of gastric mucus and bicarbonate, thus protecting the stomach and duodenal lining. It is used to treat heartburn, acid reflux, bacterial and viral infections [40] and due to its ability to stimulate new cell growth it is used in healing some types of ulcers. To reap the full benefits of DGL the tablets must be chewed and swallowed without any liquid. I used, and still do, one to two tablets 30 minutes before each meal.

2. *Herbal teas* – there is little evidence to support the beneficial effect of herbal teas on our health, even though herbs have been used for centuries for healing purposes. However, there are some herbal teas that may bring you the soothing you need when having a flare or stomach pain or acid reflux. When the GI doctor in Mexico told me I had Barrett's

esophagus and to start taking PPIs for life, I read a lot of articles on this disease to familiarize myself on what it is and what I can do to heal myself. I also investigated the natural remedies that I could take and that I used when I phased off of the PPIs in 2016. Here are some that I found useful:

a. **Slippery Elm** – contains biochemical compounds like mucilage, tannins, fatty acids. The mucilage found in the bark of slippery elm trees is a soluble fiber that forms a thick, sticky gel when in contact with water. This gel has a soothing effect and more importantly provides a protective coating on the surface of an irritated and inflamed tissue like esophagus, stomach and intestines. At the same time, the tannins and fatty acids found in its bark confer antioxidant and anti-inflammatory benefits. I used it in powder form to make teas taking advantage of the protective coating of the gel. I mixed half a teaspoon of slippery elm powder with one cup of hot water and let it steep for 5 minutes. The mixture will thicken slightly, and I was drinking it half an hour before a meal. I normally make a tea using a combination of all the ingredients I mention in this section.

b. **Marshmallow root** – the root of the marshmallow plant and its medical benefits have been known since antiquity. The benefits of drinking marshmallow root tea are related to the root's antioxidant and anti-inflammatory compounds: lowering inflammation, reducing joint pain, amongst others. The dried root has mucilage that makes it a perfect option for using it as a protective coating for the gastrointestinal tract. To use it I pour 1 cup of warm water over 1 tbsp of marshmallow root, cover it and let it sit overnight. I strain the liquid and drink it the next day 30 minutes before a meal.

c. **Licorice root** – this is a miracle plant that has been used for thousands of years to treat many health issues including fighting infections, healing stomach ulcers and other gastrointestinal problems. However, it's important to distinguish between licorice root and DGL. The former contains glycyrrhizin and can cause side effects if taken in large amounts or over a long period. That is why I preferred to take more DGL.

    d. **Ginger** - is known for its gastrointestinal soothing properties.

    e. **Chamomile and Peppermint Tea** -May help soothe the digestive tract and reduce symptoms of acid reflux. Note: Peppermint can relax the LES in some people, exacerbating reflux.

3. *Diet* – I cannot stress (nice choice of words ☺) enough the importance of a good and balanced diet on the prevention of diseases and on bringing whatever current health problems you have into remission. There are different diet choices that we will discuss more in detail in Part IV of this book with recipes of the AIP (Autoimmune Protocol Diet) in Part V. In 2011 when I was first starting the treatment with PPI after searching what to eliminate from my diet for a high stomach acid producing Barrett's esophagus I removed completely tomatoes, peppers of all kind, citric fruits, onion and garlic and I tried to eat as much as possible food with a pH greater than 5 like asparagus, beets, broccoli, cabbage, carrots, cauliflower, celery, eggplant, lettuce and so on.

Here are some suggestions:

- Avoid trigger foods, common triggers include spicy foods, citrus fruits, tomatoes, onions, garlic, fatty foods, chocolate, caffeine, and carbonated beverages.

- Eat smaller meals, larger meals can increase stomach pressure and lead to reflux. Smaller, more frequent meals can help.

- Limit alcohol and caffeine, both can relax the lower esophageal sphincter (LES), allowing stomach acid to reflux into the esophagus.

- Dietary needs and responses can be highly individual. What works for one person may not work for another, and dietary changes should ideally be made under the guidance of a nutritionist or healthcare provider.

4. *Alkaline water* - Alkaline water has been discussed as a potential aid in managing acid reflux, primarily due to its higher pH level compared to regular drinking water. Alkaline water typically has a pH above 7, which means it is less acidic than regular tap water. The premise is that by consuming a liquid with a higher pH, it may help neutralize stomach acid, thereby reducing the symptoms of acid reflux. When you drink alkaline water, it may temporarily raise the pH of your stomach. In theory, a less acidic environment in the stomach could reduce the discomfort associated with acid reflux, such as heartburn. Some studies suggest that alkaline water might be beneficial in deactivating pepsin, an enzyme involved in breaking down food proteins and a major cause of acid reflux. If alkaline water can indeed neutralize pepsin, it could potentially reduce acid reflux symptoms. Proper hydration is essential for good digestion. Drinking alkaline water can contribute to overall hydration, which is beneficial for digestive health. Well-hydrated bodies are better equipped to handle digestion and may have fewer instances of acid reflux.

5. *Other complementary approaches:* baking soda dissolved in water, magnesium carbonate dissolved in water, aloe vera juice, diluted amount of apple cider vinegar (careful since it might worsen the symptoms for some people).

In addition to all the above options to use when there is a flare in stomach acid there are some important steps to take with respect to lifestyle and stress management:

- **Lifestyle Modifications:**
    - Weight Management: Excess weight can put pressure on the abdomen, pushing stomach contents into the esophagus.
    - Elevate the Head During Sleep: Elevating the head of the bed by about 6-8 inches can help prevent acid reflux at night.
    - Avoid Lying Down After Eating: Stay upright for at least

2-3 hours after meals to allow gravity to keep acid in the stomach.

- o Quit Smoking: Smoking can weaken the LES and stimulate acid production.
- **Stress Management:**
  - o Mindfulness and Relaxation Techniques: Practices like yoga, meditation, and deep breathing can reduce stress, which may exacerbate reflux symptoms.
  - o Regular Exercise: Moderate exercise can help reduce stress and maintain a healthy weight.

2.5.3 WHY DO WE NEED STOMACH ACID?

Often, the approach in healthcare can appear to focus on diagnosing conditions and prescribing medications as a primary form of treatment. In cases where patients continue to experience symptoms, the strategy may involve identifying additional conditions and expanding the range of medications to address them.

In my career as an engineer, I've progressed through various roles, from being an engineer to a manager, and eventually, a director. My work has spanned a diverse range of design fields, including the design of linear and rotative transducers, various mechanical equipment, appliances and even skating equipment. In engineering, particularly in design, a crucial step in any new or modified project is conducting a Failure Mode Effects Analysis (FMEA). This systematic process is key to identifying potential failures in a design or manufacturing process. Through FMEA, we pinpoint potential failures, assess their implications, and prioritize them based on the severity of their consequences, their likelihood of occurrence, and the ease with which they can be detected. This analysis plays a vital role not only in mitigating risks during the design phase but also in ensuring the safety and reliability of the product before starting production or implementing any new or altered designs.

Why do I mention this?

FMEA, developed in the 1940s and applicable across various fields, raises the question of its use in evaluating the risks of acid-suppressing medications like PPIs and H2-blockers. Given the long-understood importance of stomach acid for health, it's curious whether the medical industry has fully considered the long-term risks of these drugs, such as achlorhydria. The push to market these drugs might have overshadowed thorough risk assessments, possibly due to corporate interests. Ideally, assessing these risks would require a multidisciplinary medical team, encompassing specialties like gastroenterology and endocrinology, to bring a comprehensive perspective. My own attempt at an FMEA, despite my non-medical expertise, aimed to logically and systematically analyze the potential risks of prolonged use of acid-suppressing medications, hinting at the possibility of serious chronic conditions.

Following a good FMEA practice I started by doing a very simplified flowchart of what is the role of the stomach acid, why and what is stimulating its secretion from the moment we think of food until the food passes from the stomach into the small intestine.

So, let's dive into my understanding of how our GI system works and at the end I'll talk about the FMEA analysis I did.

Before delving deeper, let's understand the basics of acidic and alkaline solutions in terms of the pH scale. This scale, which ranges from 1 to 14, is a logarithmic measure used to indicate how acidic or basic a solution is. Solutions with a pH lower than 7 are considered acidic, while those with a pH above 7 are alkaline or basic. The midpoint of the scale, pH 7, is neutral, signifying neither acidic nor alkaline. This is the typical pH level of most tap water. Interestingly, the human blood also maintains a slightly alkaline range, optimally between 7.35 and 7.45, crucial for various bodily functions [41].

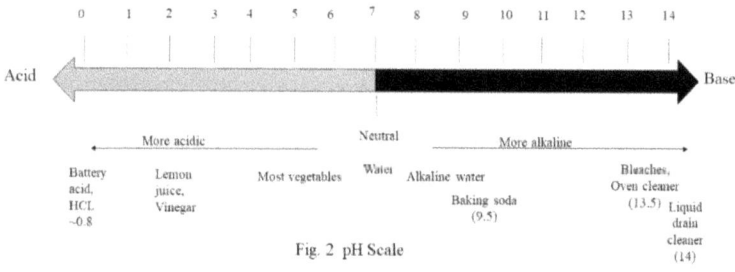

Fig. 2 pH Scale

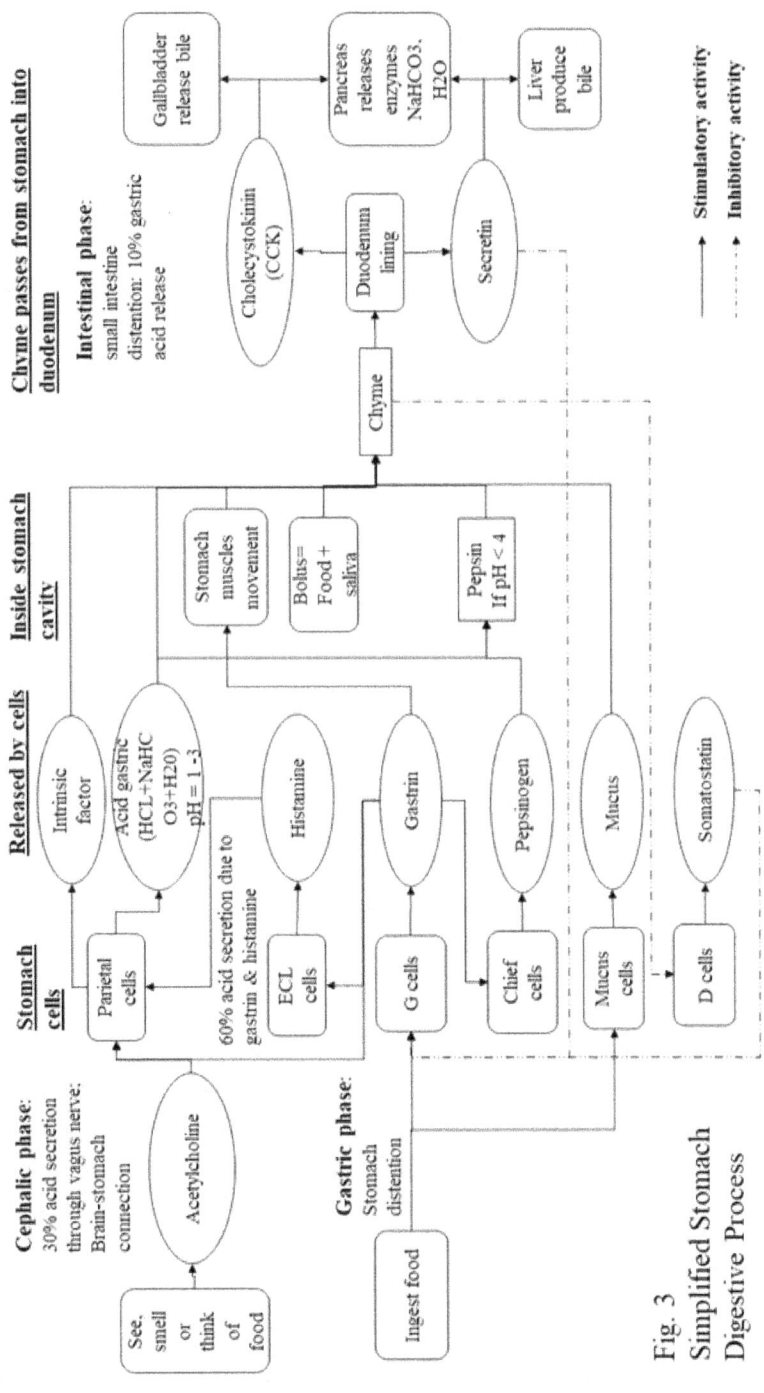

Fig. 3
Simplified Stomach Digestive Process

2.5.3.1 MY UNDERSTANDING OF WHAT HAPPENS IN OUR STOMACH AND BEYOND

> The intricacy of the human body is unparalleled. With each new discovery, our understanding deepens, and we grow more in awe of its remarkable complexity.

At the beginning of 2020, when I first suspected that I might be suffering from autoimmune gastritis, I grew increasingly curious about gastroenterologists' knowledge and their interpretations. This led me to embark on a journey of self-education, diving into various books and studies on Pernicious anemia, Hashimoto's, Autoimmune Gastritis, and autoimmune diseases more broadly. The reason for this deep dive was rooted in the understanding that one autoimmune condition often paves the way for others, due to an overactive immune system [1]. Prior to starting PPI treatment, I had been relatively healthy, which further fueled my quest to comprehend the broader impacts of acid-reducing medications on our health. To better grasp how antacids and acid suppressors' function, I developed a simplified flowchart depicting the stomach's activities from the moment we perceive food through our senses until the chyme enters the duodenum. Figure 3 in my book provides a visual representation of this process, based on my understanding of the stomach's primary activities.

From my understanding, gastric acid secretion is a complex process influenced by stimuli from the brain, stomach, and small intestine, each capable of activating or inhibiting acid production.

Here is a summarized explanation of what is happening in the digestive system [42, 43]:

- **The Cephalic phase** is brain-initiated, triggered by the mere sight, smell, or thought of an appetizing food. This phase involves the vagus nerve signaling the stomach to prepare for digestion.

- **The Gastric phase** is the stomach stimulation for acid secretion and it lasts three to four hours, depending on the type and the quantity of food we eat. Since the acid-reducer medication is acting on the H2 receptors in the case of H2-blocker medication or on the proton pump activity of the parietal cells in the case of the PPIs, I concentrated my studies on this phase, and I will explain it more in details:

  a. This phase starts the moment the food enters the stomach, and it creates a stomach distention which stimulates stomach's **G cells**.

  b. The G cells secrete a hormone, gastrin which in turn, stimulates on one side, directly the stomach's parietal cells to increase the production of HCL and on the other side stimulates the **enterochromaffin-like cells (ECL)** to secrete *histamine*.

  c. Histamine also stimulates the release of HCL by binding to the H2 receptors found in the parietal cells. This is the most important action on the parietal cells for the release of the gastric acid. The HCL mixture in the stomach, called gastric acid, has a pH between 1 and 3. An adult secretes around 1.5 liters of gastric acid each day [44].

  d. At the same time with secreting acid, the parietal cells secrete a glycoprotein called *intrinsic factor* which is of vital importance for the assimilation of vitamin B12.

  e. Simultaneously, gastrin stimulates the stomach's **chief cells** to secrete a zymogen called *pepsinogen* which in the presence of the gastric acid, it converts into an enzyme known as *pepsin*. Pepsin breaks down the proteins from food into smaller substances called peptides being very important in the protein digestion. Pepsin is produced only in an acid environment with a pH lower than 4, being more active at pH of 1.5 to 2.5. At pH higher than 5 (low acidic environment), pepsin is reversibly inactive and becomes irreversibly inactivated at pH higher than 7 [45, 46].

f. Concurrently, the stomach muscles start relaxing and contracting, pushing the bolus (food mixture with saliva) from the upper part of the stomach towards the duodenum, mixing the food with the secretions from the stomach cells. The result is called chyme. This process takes longer or shorter time, depending on the food we eat: fats take the longest time to digest, followed by proteins and then by carbohydrates [47]. Most of the food is less acidic with a pH between 4 and 7 (see table 1) [48] so as the gastric pH rises above 3 and become less acidic, the G cells secrete more gastrin which in turn stimulate the parietal cells to secrete more HCL into the stomach controlling thus the pH between 1 and 3 during the whole digestion process.

g. When the chyme, pushed by the stomach muscles, reaches the pylorus part of the stomach and a certain acidic level, the D cells start secreting Somatostatin, hormone that sends message to the G cells to slow down the secretion of gastrin and implicit of histamine by the ECL cells and finally, of HCL by the parietal cells, preparing the food mixture for the lower acidic intestinal environment.

- The Intestinal phase starts when the chyme enters the duodenum. This phase is equally important for me to study for the correct functioning of the pancreas and the gallbladder, even more so since I had to remove my gallbladder in January 2020 since it did not contract anymore to release the bile into the duodenum.

a. When the acidic chyme gets in contact with the duodenum lining it has a low pH between 2 and 4.5. This low acidic chyme activates the duodenum pH sensitive cells which in turn stimulate the intestinal S cells to secrete a hormone called secretin. This, in turn, stimulates the pancreas to secrete ions of bicarbonate (-HCO3), water and enzymes. The bicarbonate is neutralizing the pH in duodenum preparing the chyme for the small intestine where the pH is between 6 and 8 and preparing the environment for the enzymes to further break down the macronutrients from food. If the pH of the chime in the duodenum is above 4.5 the secretin cannot be released [49, 50].

b. Simultaneously with the secretion of secretin, the duodenum cells secrete cholecystokinin (CCK), a hormone that activates the gallbladder contractions to release the bile. The bile is very important in breaking down fat from food, it aids digestion and liver detoxification.

It is complicated, isn't it?

And to think that this is only a very simplified explanation of what is happening in our gastrointestinal system from the moment we ingest food until the mixture of food, enzymes and acid enters the duodenum. The whole process is much more complex than what I described above. Reading and learning all this gave me a different perspective and helped me realize what a perfectly designed mechanism we are and what poor care we take of ourselves. We actually take better care of our cars by changing the oil, regularly washing and waxing them and filling them in with high octane gas than we pay attention to our bodies' health.

pH Values of Different Common Ingredients [43]

"Variation exists between varieties, conditions of growing and processing methods"

Item	Approx. pH	Item	Approx. pH
Apple, fresh	3.2-3.9	Mushrooms	6.00-6.70
Apricots	3.30-4.80	Nectarines	3.92-4.18
Artichokes	5.50-6.00	Olives, black	6.00-7.00
Asparagus	6.00-6.70	Onions	5.3-5.8
Avocados	6.27-6.58	Oranges	3.69-4.34
Beets	5.30-6.60	Orange juice	3.30-4.19
Blueberries	3.11-3.33	Parsnip	5.30-5.70
Broccoli, cooked	6.30-6.52	Peaches	3.30-4.05
Brussels sprout	6.00-6.30	Pears, Bartlett	3.50-4.60
Cabbage, green	5.50-6.75	Peas, Garbanzo	6.48-6.80
Cantaloupe	6.13-6.58	Peppers, green	5.20-5.93
Carrots	5.88-6.40	Pineapple	3.20-4.00
Cauliflower	5.6	Plums	2.8-4.3
Celery	5.70-6.00	Pomegranate	2.93-3.20
Cherries	3.2-4.5	Potatoes	5.40-5.90
Cucumbers	5.12-5.78	Prunes	3.63-3.92
Eggplant	4.5-5.3	Pumpkin	4.990-5.50
Figs	5.05-5.98	Raspberries	3.22-3.95
Grapes	2.8-3.8	Sauerkraut	3.30-3.60
Grapefruit	3-3.7	Spinach	5.50-6.80
Leeks	5.50-6.17	Strawberries	3.00-3.90
Lemon juice	2.00-2.60	Sweet potatoes	5.30-5.60
Lime juice	2.00-2.35	Tomatoes	4.30-4.90
Mangoes, ripe	5.80-6.00	Vinegar	2.40-3.40
Mangoes, green	3.40-4.80	Vinegar, cider	3.1
Maple syrup	5.15	Watermelon	5.18-5.60
Melon, Honey dew	6.00-6.67	Zucchini	5.69-6.10

Table 1 – pH Value of Different Common Ingredients

2.5.3.2 LOW STOMACH ACID AND AUTOIMMUNE DISEASES

Stomach acid plays a crucial role in digestion and disease prevention; it not only facilitates the breakdown of food for nutrient absorption but also acts as a barrier, killing harmful bacteria and viruses that enter the stomach, thereby protecting the body from infections. Reducing stomach acid with antacid medication can inadvertently disrupt the digestive process and weaken the body's natural defense mechanism against ingested pathogens, potentially leading to chronic diseases.

Relying solely on treating the symptoms of an ailment, with limited exploration of its underlying causes, can have unfortunate consequences for patients. This approach, often observed in allopathic medicine, might inadvertently benefit pharmaceutical companies more than patients due to its focus on symptom suppression. While it's crucial to manage symptoms, true healing necessitates addressing the root causes of diseases. Until we eliminate the cause of the disease we do not cure it. The medical system, though varied in its practices, faces the challenge of balancing immediate symptom relief with long-term health solutions. Patient advocacy and informed healthcare choices play a vital role in steering towards more holistic treatment approaches.

Let's look now into what happens when we take an H2-blocker medication. As a reminder, the H-2 blockers are acid-reducers pills that attach to the parietal cells H2 receptors blocking the histamine to attach to them and to increase the HCL secretion. The H2-blockers reduce the gastric acid secretion by up to 70%.

As we can deduct from the previous chapter, our body is a perfectly "oiled" mechanism. If we do act on one of its components, we initiate a cascade effect that is affecting other parts of our body and finally, our wellbeing. In Fig. 4 you can find my interpretation of the cascading effect given by the lack of acid due to the ingestion of the H2-blocker medication.

1. **Stomach acid secretion:** The use of H2-blockers will obstruct the histamine attachment to the parietal cells' H2-receptors. The effect is a substantial reduction of the HCl secretion and therefore an increase in the stomach pH. Long-term use of H2-blockers can cause hypochlorhydria which is marked by low levels of stomach acid. A healthy person has a fasting gastric pH between 1 and 3. Fasting gastric values between 3 and 5.09 in men and 6.81 in women indicate a hypochlorhydric stomach [51, 52]. Low HCl has several important effects on the disruption of a normal functioning of our body:

    a. **Nutrient Absorption:** Vitamin and mineral deficiencies. Zinc, iron, magnesium, calcium are a few of the minerals that require stomach acid for absorption. Zinc deficiency causes low immunity, poor healing, and other conditions. Iron deficiency causes anemia, lack of energy, and immune deficiency. Vitamin B12 is also dependent on the stomach acid and the secretion of the intrinsic factor. It is vital for the nervous system and cellular function. The use of H2-blocker medication was linked to potential B12 deficiency [53]. A vitamin B12 deficiency translates into Pernicious Anemia which is an autoimmune disease. Untreated it leads to depression, extremely low energy, and neural damage.

    b. **Protein Digestion:** As indicated previously, pepsin, an essential enzyme for the protein digestion, is activated from pepsinogen and HCl if the stomach pH is at an optimum of 2 or less [45]. Maximal peptic activity is when stomach pH is between 1.5 and 2.5; when pH is between 2.5 and 5 peptic activity is reduced to approximately 70% of its maximal value and when pH ranges between 5 and 7.5 there is no pepsin activity at all, however the pepsin is stable and if the environment pH lowers to 2 the pepsin activity is restored at its maximum activity. Above environment pH of 7.5 pepsin is irreversibly inactivated [46]. This proves that in case of hypochlorhydria, when the stomach environment pH is between 3 and 5 the conversion of pepsinogen into pepsin is reduced. In addition, the activity of pepsin is reduced which translates into not all ingested food proteins (meat, eggs, nuts, seeds) will be partially broken into peptides before passing into the small intestine where they will be transformed into amino acids. This has several important effects:

i. Part of the proteins will pass into the small intestine without being broken down into amino acids. The deficiency in amino acids causes a lot of symptoms including decrease in muscle mass, extreme fatigue, difficulty concentrating, slow recovery from infections [54]. A deficiency in amino acids negatively impacts the immune system and increases the probability of acquiring a disease [55].

ii. Another effect of the proteins that are not partially digested in the stomach by pepsin is the inflammation. Only the molecules of proteins that are digested in the stomach must be absorbed in the bloodstream. The proteins not broken down into smaller blocks into the stomach are supposed to be stopped by the intestinal barrier to enter the bloodstream in the small intestine. However, due to molecular mimicry by these non-digested proteins to different molecules in our body, the breaking of the intestinal barrier allows microbes as well as undigested dietary molecules to escape the intestine into the bloodstream triggering thus an inflammatory response. This response activates chronic diseases [56]. According to studies, 80 % of people with food allergies suffer from low HCL [57]

2. Immune Function and Inflammation: Optimal stomach acid levels are vital for defending against ingested pathogens, preventing bacteria overgrowth, and supporting the immune system and decreasing the occurrence of inflammation in the body [58]. Hypochlorhydria compromises this defense mechanism, increasing susceptibility to infections and chronic

diseases. Inadequately digested proteins can also trigger inflammatory responses, contributing to chronic health issues.

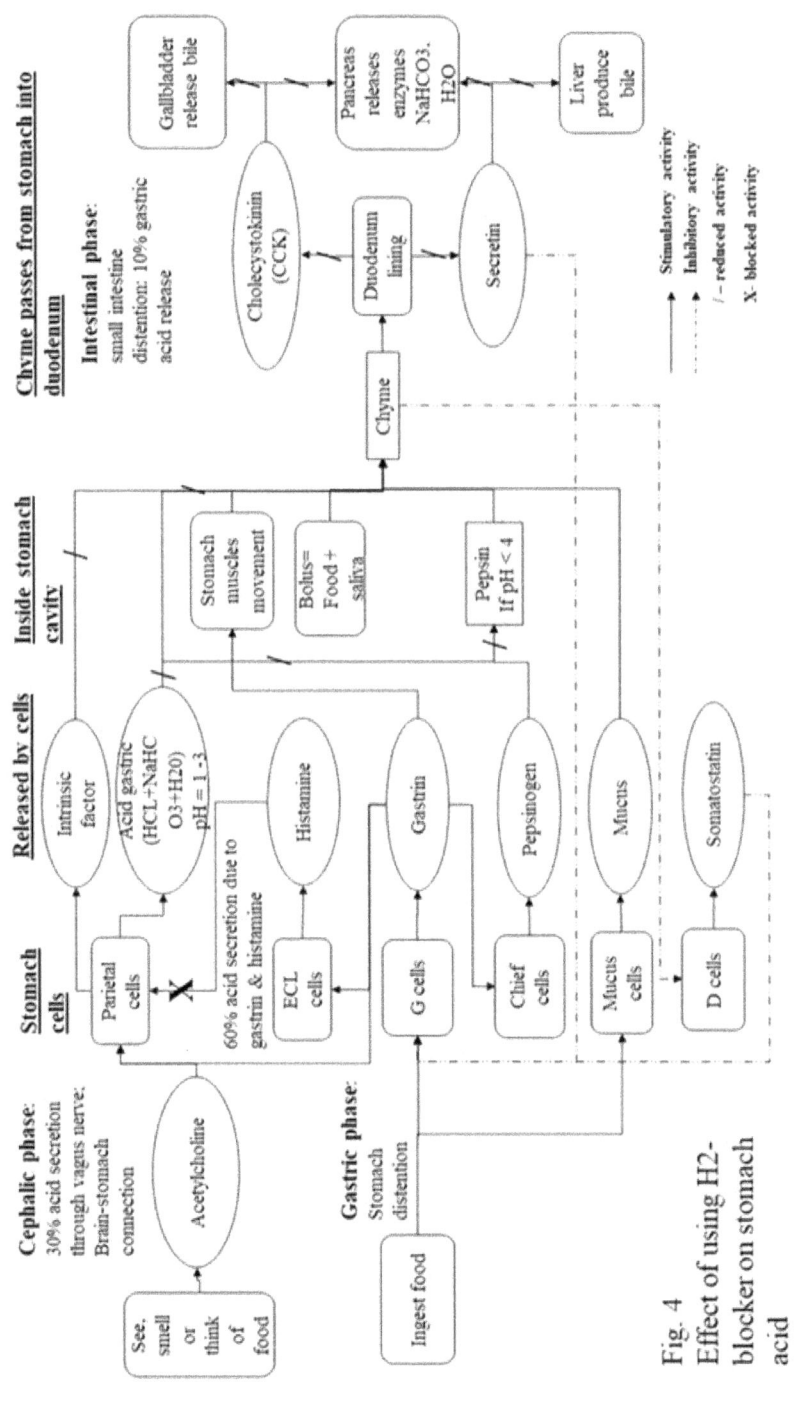

Fig. 4
Effect of using H2-blocker on stomach acid

3. **Bile and Pancreas Function**: In a healthy person the chime that passes from the stomach into the intestine must have a pH of around 2. By using H2-blocker medication the pH in the stomach increases between 3 and 5, however, most of the food we eat has a pH above 5. This makes the chyme, which is the mixture of food, saliva, stomach enzymes, mucus and HCl, have a pH above 5 as well, or, in the best scenario, if we eat something acidic like grapefruit, oranges, plums, the chyme pH could be below 4. At the same time, the protein and the fat in food are not properly digested in the stomach. There are several implications of a chyme with higher pH (not too acidic) entering the duodenum and inhibiting the release of secretin and cholecystokinin.

   a. The secretin is released optimally only if the pH in the duodenum is below 4.5. As a result of a chyme with higher pH, secretin cannot be released, or it might be released but not in the optimal quantity. This hormone responds to the acidity of the chyme, and it stimulates the secretion of the bile in the liver. Not having enough HCL, the secretin secretion being hindered, it might not stimulate the bile secretion from the gallbladder. Studies "indicate that the recent rise in use of [stomach] acid-suppressing medications might have contributed to the increased incidence of chronic liver disease" [59]. The flow of bile is one of the liver's most important elimination routes for toxins. When bile flow into the intestines is reduced, it can lead to bacterial infections [54].

   b. Cholecystokinin, secreted by the small intestine in response to fats and amino acids in chyme, plays a key role in stimulating the pancreas and gallbladder. It prompts the release of pancreatic enzymes and the contraction of the gallbladder, facilitating bile flow into the duodenum for fat digestion. A less acidic stomach means a less effective nutrient breakdown and therefore less stimulation of the gallbladder due to less cholecystokinin secretion. This can lead to a sluggish gallbladder which in turn disrupts the detoxification of the liver and to cholesterol imbalances. Bile flow in the gastrointestinal tract is essential in preventing infections of pathogenic bacteria [60].

The above description of the effects of the H2-blocker medication is very simplified but the effects are very serious and can diminish the quality of life due to the serious symptoms related to the lack of HCl secretion.

The action of the PPI medication is similar, but the effects are more severe and that is mainly due to the fact that the H2-blocker drugs stop only one branch of the production of HCl in the stomach as you can see in Fig. 4, that is by blocking the action of histamine at the histamine H2 receptors in the parietal cells in the stomach, while the PPI medication goes directly to the source of the acid production and inhibits the HCl secretion directly at the proton pump activity of the parietal cells. That is why the PPI medication prevents up to 95% of acid production which brings us to a state of achlorhydria defined by "an intragastric pH greater than 5.09 in men and greater than 6.81 in women." (57, 58).

In Fig. 5 I show my interpretation of the impact of taking PPI medication on the acid and enzyme secretion in the stomach and the duodenum. Since the stomach pH is higher (achlorhydria) when taking PPIs the cascading effect of the lack of acid is more accentuated:

1. **Acid secretion:** Fasting gastric values are above 5.09 in men and 6.81 in women which indicate an achlorhydric stomach [61]. All side effects of the lack of acid discussed previously are seen when taking PPIs as well:

    a. **Nutrient Absorption:** Vitamins and mineral deficiencies may lead to autoimmune diseases. Vitamin B12 not being absorbed due to the intrinsic factor not being secreted will lead to Pernicious anemia which can be fatal if not discovered and treated accordingly [62].

    b. **Protein Digestion:** Pepsin is not created in absence of HCl and the food and proteins will not be broken into smaller particles ready to be digested furthermore in the small intestine. This may lead to amino acids deficiency and inflammation.

   c. **Immune and Inflammation:** Lack of HCl will not destroy bacteria, viruses, parasites that enter the digestive tract through food or drinks, leaving our body open to infections. The protective barrier of HCl being broken can damage the gut and lead to digestive and health issues. Bacteria may develop in the small intestine forcing the immune system to overreact and possibly to attack the body's own molecules to get rid of the intruders.

2. **Bile and Pancreas Function:** The chyme has a pH close to the neutral 7 and will not activate the pancreas and liver enzymes. The gallbladder will not be stimulated to contract and release the bile into the small intestine. In addition to undigested food, nutrients malabsorption and bacteria overgrowth the effect is also a poor pancreas functioning, accumulation of toxins in the liver and body, high cholesterol and potentially gallbladder removal. I did experience the above symptoms, the removal of the gallbladder due to not releasing the bile in the duodenum and my cholesterol is high despite my very clean lifestyle and eating habits.

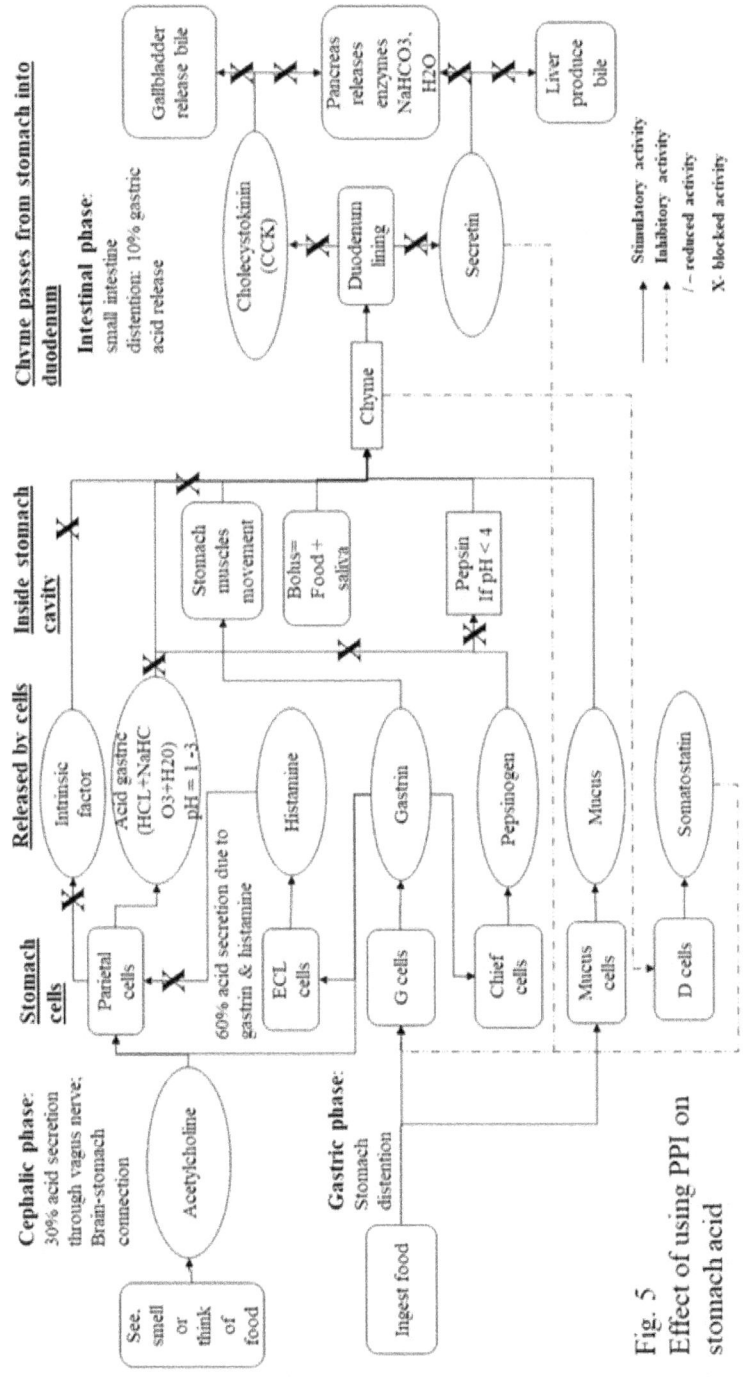

Fig. 5
Effect of using PPI on stomach acid

Symptoms of hypochlorhydria or achlorhydria are [63]:

- **Feeling too full after meals:** Common in hypochlorhydria, as reduced acid can slow digestion.
- **Indigestion:** A core symptom, resulting from impaired food breakdown.
- **Gas and Bloating:** Often occurs due to fermentation of undigested food by bacteria in the gut.
- **Diarrhea and Constipation:** Digestive irregularities are common with altered gastric acid.
- **Stomach upset (dyspepsia) or cramps:** Typical symptoms due to indigestion.
- **Undigested food in stool:** Indicates poor digestion, often due to inadequate acid levels.
- **Nausea:** Can occur due to accumulation of undigested food in the stomach.
- **Heartburn:** Paradoxically, low stomach acid can cause symptoms similar to excess acid.
- **Epigastric pain:** Pain in the upper stomach region is common with digestive disorders.
- **Acid regurgitation:** Can occur even with low acid levels, often due to impaired gastric function.
- **Early satiety:** Feeling full quickly may be due to slower digestion and gastric emptying.
- **Dysphagia (difficulty swallowing):** Less common but can occur if gastric issues affect esophageal function.
- **Abdominal discomfort:** A general symptom associated with many digestive conditions, including hypochlorhydria.

If the low stomach acid persists for a longer period, chances of developing iron anemia, pernicious anemia, Hashimoto's, or autoimmune gastritis are increasing. Some symptoms related to these diseases, in addition to those above are [64]:

- **Trouble Digesting Meat or Vegetables:** Can occur in autoimmune gastritis and anemias due to reduced stomach acid affecting protein digestion.

- **Bacterial Infections:** More common in cases of reduced stomach acid (as in autoimmune gastritis) which normally helps eliminate harmful bacteria.

- **Fatigue:** A key symptom of both iron and pernicious anemia, and commonly reported in Hashimoto's and other autoimmune conditions.

- **Joint Inflammation:** Often associated with autoimmune diseases, where the immune system attacks joint tissues.

- **Brain Fog:** Common in Hashimoto's due to thyroid hormone imbalances and in anemias due to reduced oxygen supply to the brain.

- **Acid Reflux:** Can be a symptom of autoimmune gastritis and other gastrointestinal autoimmune disorders.

- **Weakness:** Often results from the fatigue and nutrient deficiencies seen in anemias and autoimmune diseases.

- **Pain:** A broad symptom that can be present in many autoimmune diseases due to inflammation and tissue damage.

- **Food Allergies:** Increased in autoimmune diseases due to altered immune responses.

- **Asthma:** There is a potential link between autoimmune activity and asthma, although the relationship is complex.

- **Skin Problems (Acne, Psoriasis, Rosacea):** Skin conditions like psoriasis are autoimmune in nature, and autoimmune activity can exacerbate acne and rosacea.

- **Weak and Brittle Nails, Hair Loss:** Common in thyroid disorders like Hashimoto's and in iron deficiency anemia.

- **Depression:** Often associated with autoimmune diseases and anemias, possibly due to physiological stress and nutrient deficiencies.

- **Reduced Ability to Concentrate:** A symptom commonly reported in Hashimoto's thyroiditis and anemia.

- **Insomnia:** Can occur in autoimmune diseases, including Hashimoto's, often due to discomfort, pain, or hormonal imbalances.

If having some of the above symptoms is a concern, there are tests that can confirm stomach low acid [61, 63]:

- **Parietal Cell Antibodies Test:** Used to detect the presence of antibodies against gastric parietal cells. This test can help diagnose autoimmune gastritis, a condition that can lead to low stomach acid.

- **Intrinsic Factor Antibody Test:** Intrinsic factor is crucial for vitamin B12 absorption. Antibodies against it can indicate pernicious anemia, which is often associated with reduced stomach acid.

- **Endoscopy with Stomach Biopsy:** An endoscopic examination allows direct visualization of the stomach lining and the collection of tissue samples (biopsies). This can help identify gastritis, cellular changes, and potential causes of low acid production.

- **Gastric pH Monitoring:** Directly measures the pH level within the stomach. This is a definitive way to assess the level of stomach acidity.

- **Serum Gastrin Test:** Gastrin is a hormone that stimulates stomach acid production. Elevated levels can indicate a compensatory response to low stomach acid or other related conditions.

- **Serum Pepsinogen Test:** Pepsinogen is a precursor to pepsin, an enzyme important in protein digestion. Low levels can be indicative of atrophic gastritis, a condition that reduces stomach acid production.

- **Hemoglobin Level:** Part of a complete blood count (CBC), used to detect anemia, which can be a consequence of chronic gastritis or B12 deficiency due to low stomach acid.

- **Stool Test for H. pylori and Bacterial Overgrowth Infections:** H. pylori is a bacterium that can cause gastritis and ulcers, leading to changes in stomach acid production. Testing for bacterial overgrowth is also important, as low stomach acid can predispose to increased bacterial colonization in the stomach and small intestine.

Low stomach acid may be the cause of several diseases [64, 65]:

- **Acne Rosacea:** Some studies suggest a link between gastrointestinal health and skin conditions like rosacea.

- **Allergic Reactions:** Hypochlorhydria may affect gut health and immune function, potentially influencing allergic responses.

- **Chronic Autoimmune Hepatitis:** This is a liver condition, and overall digestive health can impact liver function.

- **Gallbladder Disease:** Gallbladder function and health can be influenced by digestive processes, including acid production in the stomach.

- **Graves' Disease and Hashimoto's Disease:** Both are thyroid conditions with autoimmune components and there can be interactions due to overall health and nutrient absorption.

- **Osteoporosis:** Low stomach acid can impact mineral absorption, including calcium, which is vital for bone health.

- **Pernicious Anemia:** Directly related to low stomach acid due to its impact on vitamin B12 absorption.

- **Rheumatoid Arthritis:** An autoimmune condition, where overall health, including gut health, may play a role.

- **Ulcerative Colitis:** Primarily a disease of the colon, and overall gut health, including stomach acid can play a role.

The list of potential diseases that have the cause of low stomach acid is longer. A very good book that explains very well the causes and effects of hypochlorhydria/achlorhydria is "Why stomach acid is good for you. Natural relief from Heartburn, Indigestion, Reflux & GERD" by Jonathan V. Wright, MD and Lane Lenard, Ph.D.

Unfortunately, we, humans, are sometimes the lab-rats and get sick while the pharmaceutical companies that market these drugs get richer and richer. Increasing evidence from recent studies points to potential harmful effects associated with long-term use of acid-reducing medications. Few years ago, a mass class action was issued against the manufacturers of Nexium, Prilosec, Prevacid and other PPIs for kidney injuries. There are studies that link the PPI medication to kidney stones. According to an article in Clinical Gastroenterology and Hepatology [66], "we found PPI used to be associated with a dose-dependent increase in risk of kidney stones. H2RA use also has an association with risk of kidney stones, so acid suppression might be an involved mechanism." From personal experience, the frequency of my kidney stones increased significantly—from one every 10-15 years to one every 3-4 years—after starting PPI medication.

A study conducted on the effects of Proton Pump Inhibitors (PPIs) on the gut microbiome assessed the gut microbiome composition of 1,815 individuals across three cohorts. The study found that PPI use is associated with a significant decrease in the diversity of the gut microbiome and changes in 20% of the bacterial categories. The study concluded that PPI use leads to changes in the gut microbiome towards a less healthy state, which aligns with the known predisposition to Clostridium difficile infections. It was noted that the impact of PPIs on the gut microbiome is more significant than the effects of antibiotics or other commonly used drugs [5].

Gut dysbiosis, also known as intestinal dysbiosis, is a condition where there's an imbalance in the gut microbiota, which is the community of microorganisms, including both beneficial and harmful bacteria, that inhabit the digestive tract. The human microbiota consists of trillions of these microorganisms, with bacteria, fungi, and others predominantly residing in the colon, particularly in the jejunum and ileum sections. The two dominant bacterial strains in a healthy gut are Firmicutes and Bacteroides.

These microbes are crucial for various aspects of health. They play an integral role in digestion, aiding in the absorption of essential minerals and vitamins. Additionally, they are key contributors to immune function and metabolism and are even involved in regulating mental health. In a well-balanced gut microbiome, there is a diverse population of these beneficial microorganisms coexisting in harmony.

However, when this balance is disrupted, leading to gut dysbiosis, it can negatively affect the immune system and inflammatory responses. This imbalance may contribute to the development of autoimmune diseases, as the altered microbiome can trigger abnormal immune responses in the body. Gut dysbiosis is a significant health concern due to its potential wide-ranging effects on overall well-being [67].

Several factors can lead to an imbalance in the gut microbiota, known as gut dysbiosis. Here are some common causes:

- **Acid-Reducing Medications:** Medications like Proton Pump Inhibitors (PPIs) and H2-blockers reduce stomach acid, which can lead to increased gut permeability, Small Intestine Bacterial Overgrowth (SIBO), an overactive immune system, and potentially, autoimmune diseases.

- **Antibiotic Use:** Antibiotics can disrupt the balance of gut microbiota by eliminating both harmful and beneficial bacteria.

- **Chronic Stress:** Long-term stress can affect the gut-brain axis, altering the composition of the gut microbiota.

- **Infections:** Certain infections can cause dysbiosis, upsetting the balance of gut bacteria.

- Environmental Factors: Exposure to certain toxins or pollutants can have adverse effects on the gut microbiota.

Gut dysbiosis, or the imbalance in the gut microbiota, can lead to significant health issues, including:

- **Digestive Problems:** Common symptoms such as bloating, gas, and diarrhea can be direct consequences of gut dysbiosis, as the imbalance affects digestive processes.

- **Immune System Dysfunction:** The gut microbiota is instrumental in regulating immune system homeostasis and the development of immune cells. Approximately 70% of the entire immune system is in the gut-associated lymphoid tissue (GALT), where the gut microbiome plays a critical role. Dysbiosis can lead to immune system dysregulation, increasing vulnerability to infections and autoimmune diseases.

- **Chronic Low-Level Inflammation:** Many autoimmune conditions are associated with or exacerbated by chronic inflammation, which can be a byproduct of gut dysbiosis.

- **Mental Health Effects:** The gut-brain axis, which connects the gut and the brain, suggests that gut dysbiosis can influence mental health. This connection underscores the importance of a balanced gut microbiome for overall psychological well-being.

The analysis and management of gut dysbiosis, which can be the underlying cause of various diseases and symptoms, requires a comprehensive approach beyond just taking probiotics and prebiotics. It's crucial to address the root cause of dysbiosis. For instance, if gut dysbiosis is due to the prolonged use of Proton Pump Inhibitors (PPIs) leading to reduced stomach acid, simply supplementing with probiotics/prebiotics may not suffice. In such cases, discontinuing PPIs and possibly supplementing with Hydrochloric Acid (HCl) may be necessary to restore gut health.

For those currently on H2-blocker or PPI medication, it is important not to discontinue these drugs abruptly without consulting a healthcare provider. If concerns persist regarding the use of these medications, seeking the advice of a Functional Medicine doctor can be beneficial, as they often adopt a more holistic approach to treatment.

Additionally, if you are not currently taking acid-suppressing medication but your doctor is considering prescribing it for heartburn or GERD based solely on symptoms, requesting a gastric pH monitoring test can provide a clearer understanding of whether excess stomach acid is actually the issue. This test can help in making more informed decisions about appropriate treatment options.

Undertaking a comprehensive analysis of stomach acid's role and its suppression effects, as well as creating flowcharts to simplify this understanding, sets a solid foundation for delving into a Failure Mode Effects Analysis (FMEA) study. Remember, FMEA is a proactive approach used at the initial stages of a design process, including drug development, to identify and mitigate potential risks associated with a new design or product.

In the context of pharmaceuticals, an FMEA study is particularly crucial for new medications. This analysis aims to foresee and address potential serious side effects that could pose risks to patient health. By conducting an FMEA, pharmaceutical companies can assess the safety and efficacy of a drug before it reaches the market, ensuring that any significant risks are identified, and strategies are developed to mitigate them. This process is essential for safeguarding patient health and improving the overall quality and safety of pharmaceutical products.

Prolonged use (exceeding eight weeks) of acid-suppression medication, such as H2-blockers and Proton Pump Inhibitors (PPIs), may be associated with the development of irreversible chronic autoimmune diseases [68]. While the exact causes of many autoimmune diseases remain elusive, one contributing factor is increasingly recognized: the reduction of stomach acid due to long-term use of acid-suppressing medication.

Doctors have a responsibility to clearly communicate the risks and benefits of any medication to their patients. It's crucial that patients are involved in the decision-making process regarding their treatment. For medications as potent as acid-suppressors, prescribing them should ideally follow thorough diagnostic procedures, such as gastric pH testing, rather than solely relying on symptom-based assessments and assumptions about excessive stomach acid. Ensuring a more precise diagnosis can help in making more informed decisions about the necessity and duration of using acid-suppression medication.

With a comprehensive understanding of stomach acid's crucial role in food digestion and maintaining a healthy microbiome, we can explore whether an FMEA (Failure Mode and Effects Analysis) could predict the significant impacts of acid-suppressing medications on health. FMEA is a systematic approach used to identify and address potential failures in a design—in this case, the design being the acid-suppressing medication and its effects on user health. This process ideally involves a multidisciplinary team including gastroenterologists, hematologists, endocrinologists, and urologists to thoroughly assess the broad implications of altering stomach acid levels. The analysis requires assigning a severity ranking to each potential failure effect, such as those resulting from hypochlorhydria (low stomach acid) or achlorhydria (no stomach acid) and quantifying their impact on health using a predefined scale and rules.

Severity of Failure	No effect (Failure is not noticeable and does not affect the patient's health)	1
	Slight effect (Failure causes minor effects or is a minor trouble to the patient)	3
	Moderate effect (Failure causes some performance loss))	5
	Major effect (Failure causes a high degree of performance loss, with permanent impact on the health of the patient)	7
	Severe or catastrophic effect (Failure causes death or major, permanent loss of function)	#

Likelihood of occurrence	3 months	1
	3 months to 1 year	5
	1-3 yrs	10

Assigning an occurrence ranking for each potential failure from acid-suppressing medications, like H2-blockers or PPIs, which can reduce stomach acid by up to 70% and 95% respectively, is challenging. The key question in determining this ranking is how quickly the effects of such significant acid reduction can be detected. Estimating the time it takes for diseases caused by the lack of stomach acid to manifest is complex. Although I have created a scale to assess the likelihood of these occurrences, for this analysis, I've assumed that effects of having low stomach acid (such as vitamin and mineral deficiencies, gut bacteria unbalances…) will manifest after more than one year of continuous medication use.

Finally, I need to assign the difficulty of detection, so the question to answer here is how easily a certain health problem attributable to the lack of stomach acid can be detected. This involves considering the diagnostic tools and methods available, as well as the subtlety or overt nature of symptoms that might arise from such conditions. Then, I'm ready to identify and record the functions of stomach acid in our body and analyze what occurs if these functions are compromised by acid-suppressing medication. Throughout this exercise, I've aimed for objectivity, drawing on knowledge from various articles and books about the significance of stomach acid. The risk priority number for each potential failure is calculated by multiplying the severity of the failure, the likelihood of its occurrence, and the difficulty of its detection. This approach helps quantify the impact of each failure on the intended function of stomach acid.

	Easy to detect early with tests	1
Difficulty of Detection	Not so easy to detect with tests but tendency in time can show deterioration	4
	Symptoms can show a problem is ongoing but it goes undetected or mistaken for other diseases	7
	Not detectable until irreversible changes occur	10

POTENTIAL FAILURE MODE EFFECT ANALYSIS

PURPOSE: Evaluate the impact of PPI medication (lower stomach acid by up to 95%) on overall health

N.O.	INTENDED FUNCTION OF STOMACH ACID	POTENTIAL FAILURE MODE	POTENTIAL FAILURE EFFECTS	SEVERITY OF FAILURE		LIKELIHOOD OF OCCURENCE		DIFFICULTY OF DETECTION	
				SF	POTENTIAL CAUSE	LO	CURRENT CONTROL EVALUATION	DD	RISK PRORITY
5	Convert pepsinogen to pepsin	Undigested proteins passing into the duodenum (51)	Neuroinflammatory diseases: - Multiple sclerosis - Alzheimer's - Parkinson's - Amyotrophic lateral sclerosis - Autism spectrum disorders Other diseases: - Autoimmune gastritis - Hashimoto's - Leaky gut - IBS, IBD	10	undigested molecules getting in the bloodstream through the intestinal mucosal due to molecular mimicry of body molecules	10	Difficult to detect proactively until the disease is set in.	10	1000
8	Partially digesting food before entering the small intestine	undigested proteins passing into the duodenum (51)	autoimmune diseases: - Autoimmune gastritis - Hashimoto's - Leaky gut - IBS, IBD	10	undigested molecules getting in the bloodstream through the intestinal mucosal due to molecular mimicry of body molecules	10	Difficult to detect until changes in the body are made and antibodies are affecting different organs.	10	1000
10	Antibacterial - Barrier agains microorganisms and infection prevention	Gut inflammation and growth of bacteria	autoimmune diseases, chronic liver disease (72)	10	gut microbiome changes due to low stomach acid	10	blood test, stool tests but lots of time can go undetected	10	1000

NO.	INTENDED FUNCTION OF STOMACH ACID	POTENTIAL FAILURE MODE	POTENTIAL FAILURE EFFECTS	SEVERITY OF FAILURE		LIKELIHOOD OF OCCURRENCE		DIFFICULTY OF DETECTION	
				POTENTIAL CAUSE	SF	CURRENT CONTROL EVALUATION	LO	RISK PRIORITY	DD
9	Antibacterial - Barrier against microorganisms and infection prevention	Bacterial overgrowth, parasites	bloating, upset stomach, diarrhea, constipation, heartburn, gas, indigestion, frequent infections, migraines, anemia, anxiety, E.coli, Streptococci, cholera dysentery, typhoid, tuberculosis, Candida yeast, Cmpylobacter pylory (48).	Gastric acid can kill bacteria within 15 min. if pH is less than 3. At pH above 4 bacteria overgrowth can occur (69)	10	blood test, stool tests	10	700	7
11	Helps the release of pancreatic enzymes in small intestine	Low pancreatic enzymes (70,71, 74)	food sensitivities acid reflux or burning bloating abdominal pain gastritis chronic gut inflammation Chron's disease Celiac disease Acute and Chronic pancreatitis Cystic fibrosis Pancreatic cancer	Low stomach acid inhibits the secretion of pancreatic enzymes	10	stool test, pancreatic function test, blood tests	10	700	7
12	Helps the release of bile in the liver and gallbladder contraction to release the bile	Low bile secretion and gallbladder contractions	diarrhea, toxic build up gallbladder stones sluggish gallbladder, fatty liver	Low stomach acid inhibits the secretion of bile (53)	10	Blood test, CT scan, MRI	10	700	7

N.O.	INTENDED FUNCTION OF STOMACH ACID	POTENTIAL FAILURE MODE	POTENTIAL FAILURE EFFECTS	SEVERITY OF FAILURE SF	POTENTIAL CAUSE	LIKELIHOOD OF OCCURENCE LO	CURRENT CONTROL EVALUATION	DD	DIFFICULTY OF DETECTION RISK PRIORITY
3	Convert pepsinogen to pepsin	At higher pH (alkaline environment) pepsinogen is not converted in pepsin. (6+). Some of all protein from food will not be broken down and properly digested in the stomach and potentially not absorbed. Pepsin needs an environment with a pH lower than 4 to be formed	fatigue, weakness	5	loss of muscle mass	10	Total protein test	7	350
4	Convert pepsinogen to pepsin	At higher pH (alkaline environment) pepsinogen is not converted in pepsin. (6+). Some of all protein from food will not be broken down and properly digested in the stomach and potentially not absorbed. Pepsin needs an environment with a pH lower than 4 to be formed	slow-healing injuries	5	collagen deficiency	10	Collagen Disorder Profile blood test	7	350
1	Convert pepsinogen to pepsin	At higher pH (alkaline environment) pepsinogen is not converted in pepsin. (6+). Some of all protein from food will not be broken down and properly digested in the stomach and potentially not absorbed. Pepsin needs an environment with a pH lower than 4 to be formed	Mood changes, depression, anxiety, maldigestion malabsorbtion, fatigue,	5	protein deficiency means amino acid defficiency which impact the neurotransmitters which may in turn affect brain functionality (serotonin, dopamine...)	10	amino acids blood tests Urine Amino Acids	4	200

N.O.	INTENDED FUNCTION OF STOMACH ACID	POTENTIAL FAILURE MODE	POTENTIAL FAILURE EFFECTS	SEVERITY OF FAILURE SF	POTENTIAL CAUSE	LIKELIHOOD OF OCCURENCE LO	CURRENT CONTROL EVALUATION	DIFFICULTY OF DETECTION DD	RISK PRORITY
2	Convert pepsinogen to pepsin	At higher pH (alkaline environment) pepsinogen is not converted in pepsin. (64). Some of all protein from food will not be broken down and properly digested in the stomach and potentially not absorbed. Pepsin needs an environment with a pH lower than 4 to be formed.	Thinning hair, brittle nails and dry skin	3	elastin, collagen, keratin deficiency	10	Total protein test	4	120
7	Partially digesting food before entering the small intestine	Vitamin and mineral deficiencies (iron, vitamin D, E, C, calcium, zinc, magnezium, selenium..) (65,66,67)	anemia, weakness, fatigue, poor concentration, osteoporosis, frequent infections, muscle cramps, hair loss, depression, weak muscles	5	vitamins, minerals, proteins and amino acids need a narrow range of pH to be absorbed (68)	10	blood tests to see minerals and vitamins tendency in time	1	50
6	Helps to release intrinsic factor	Vitamin B12 deficiency	Pernicious anemia, weakness, peripheral neuropathy, depression, myelopathy, brain fog, weakness, fatigue.	4	Parietal cells blocked to release intrinsic factor (62,63)	10	blood tests to see B12 tendency in time	1	40

The most challenging aspect in evaluating the Failure Mode Effects Analysis (FMEA) concerning stomach acid operation is determining the Difficulty of Detection (DD) for potential failures. This difficulty arises partly from my limited knowledge of all the diagnostic tests available in the medical field. A team comprising various medical specialists could more effectively identify and utilize the relevant diagnostic tests.

Moreover, even when vitamin or mineral deficiencies, such as deficiencies in Vitamins B12 and D, are easily detectable, they are often not immediately attributed to the long-term use of acid-suppressing medications like Nexium. For instance, in 2013, I was diagnosed with deficiencies in these vitamins, but no connection was made to my four years of continuous PPIs usage.

Lastly, the idea of detecting a trend towards a disease or deficiency over time, based on test results, seems theoretically sound. However, in practice, this approach has limitations. From my experience, it's rare to find healthcare providers who systematically review past test results to identify such trends. This lack of comprehensive analysis can hinder the early detection and attribution of developing health issues to specific medications.

The primary objective of this Failure Mode Effects Analysis (FMEA) is to scrutinize the consequences of reduced stomach acid, specifically stemming from the prolonged use of acid-suppressing medications. This analysis aims to assess whether the adverse effects of such medications could have been anticipated before their widespread prescription for symptoms attributed to 'excess acid.' The graphic representation of the FMEA highlights various potential failures linked to the diminished functionality of stomach acid.

Critical among these failures are those designated as numbers 1, 2, and 3. These correspond to the inability to convert pepsinogen into pepsin and to properly digest food before it enters the small intestine. Furthermore, they also represent the compromised role of stomach acid as an antibacterial barrier, potentially leading to gut inflammation and bacterial overgrowth. The risk associated with these failure modes is alarmingly high, given their direct link to the digestive process and infection prevention. Consequently, these failures could lead to the development of autoimmune diseases, underlining the significant impact of impaired stomach acid functionality.

In the realm of stomach acid suppression through medication, our analysis identifies significant risk priorities tied to numbers 4, 5, and 6. These risks are associated with the failure of stomach acid to act as an effective barrier against microorganisms, leading to bacterial overgrowth, and the subsequent failure to adequately activate pancreatic and liver enzymes. This highlights a critical concern regarding the broad implications of acid suppression on bodily functions.

To determine a threshold for risk priority, which could indicate severe illnesses or the potential development of chronic autoimmune diseases, we must scrutinize three key factors: the Difficulty of Detection, the Severity of Failure, and the Likelihood of Occurrence. For the Difficulty of Detection, I assigned a ranking of 4, suggesting that diseases stemming from reduced stomach acid due to medication use are not easily identified as being caused by an alkaline stomach environment. A pertinent example is my own experience with vitamin and mineral deficiencies, where no link was established between PPI-induced high stomach pH and malabsorption of vitamins B12 and D. In my case, the immediate response was to prescribe supplements, rather than investigate the underlying cause of the malabsorption, which was related to medication-induced changes in stomach acidity.

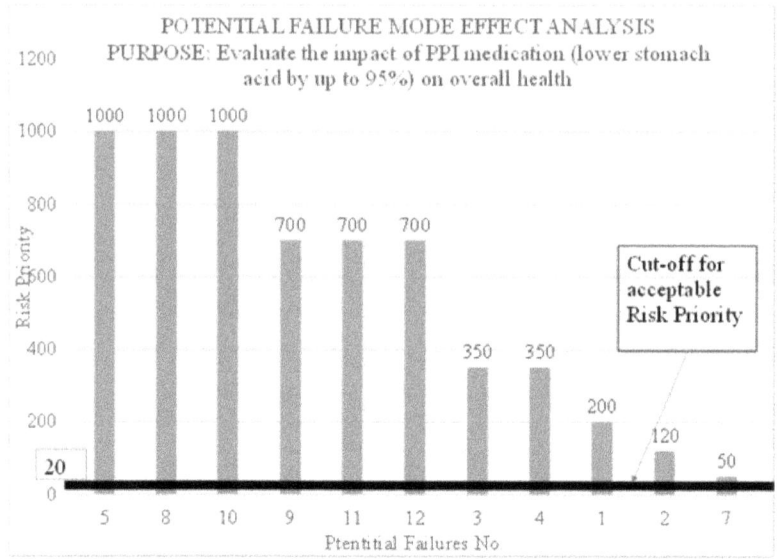

If a thorough FMEA had been conducted prior to the market release of acid-suppressing medications, a crucial risk mitigation strategy would have involved instructing prescribing physicians to monitor the trend of vitamin and mineral levels in the blood over time in patients on these drugs. This proactive approach could have potentially identified and addressed the root cause of deficiencies, rather than merely treating the symptoms with additional medication.

For the Severity of Failure ranking, I chose 5 which corresponds to a loss of performance (weakness, lack of energy, concentration, brain fog, muscles pain) which can be reversed if the PPI medication is stopped. This again requires an empathetic doctor that takes the time needed to listen to you and to believe you are not hypochondriac when explaining your symptoms as it happened to me and to a lot of other people that complained about some of these symptoms. At every yearly appointment I had with my GI for endoscopies he was pushing me to take antidepressant medication telling me that the symptoms are only in my head, and he continued to pump me (pun intended) with Proton Pump Inhibitors.

Finally, for the Likelihood of Occurrence I chose 1 since even though PPIs might prove helpful for some diseases like stomach ulcers, the healing process lasts between 4 and 6 weeks if treated with acid-reducing medication. If the drugs are taken for more than 8 weeks, then adverse effects will start manifesting. For other medical conditions for which PPIs are recommended to be taken for longer time or for life (like Barrett's esophagus) taking PPI will not solve the health problem but it will only change one disease for several others produced by the side effects of the acid-suppressing medication (Pernicious Anemia, hypomagnesemia, hypocalcemia, pneumonia, C. difficile, etc.).

Using these rankings, the Potential Risk cut-off is 20. This means that for every health failure caused by a low level of stomach acid that has a calculated Potential Risk higher than 20, the probability of developing a serious chronic or life-threatening disease due to the usage of an H2-blocker or PPI medication for longer than 3 months is very high. The higher the calculated Potential Risk, the higher the probability.

The completion of this analysis hinges on laboratory and cohort studies that will validate the effects of both short-term and long-term use of acid-suppressing drugs. Future research should focus on gathering empirical data to refine the Potential Risk assessment further.

While this Failure Mode Effects Analysis (FMEA) is a solo effort by someone outside the medical profession, its objective is to demonstrate that if a thorough and logical evaluation had been conducted by a diverse group of independent medical experts, the use of long-term acid-suppressing medication might have been restricted. Such a collaborative approach could have led to guidelines limiting the use of these drugs to no more than three months or even less for any condition. Furthermore, this precaution might have extended to preventing these medications from being available over the counter.

One of the most significant ironies highlighted by this exercise is the prevalent prescription of Proton Pump Inhibitors (PPIs) for Gastroesophageal Reflux Disease (GERD), despite many of these cases actually being characterized by low stomach acid, not high.

Every profession, whether it's engineering, technical repair, or electrical work, demands strong investigative abilities to thoroughly understand problems and devise enduring solutions. Similarly, being an effective doctor also requires these skills, along with patience, empathy, a genuine passion for the field, and logical reasoning. Without these qualities, a doctor may overlook the underlying cause of a patient's ailment. Regrettably, many individuals enter the medical profession driven by financial incentives, the prestige associated with being a doctor, or the autonomy the job offers. Often, their approach to healthcare is shaped more by the directives of influential, financially motivated entities and rule-makers than by patient-centered considerations.

The **FMEA (Failure Mode Effects Analysis) approach is adaptable and can be applied to any medication. My focus on acid-reducing drugs stems from my personal experience and extensive research into the digestive system. However, this analytical process is equally valuable for examining other types of medications.**

One key insight from this exercise is the intricate interdependence within the digestive system. A disturbance in one aspect, such as decreased stomach acid, can trigger dysfunctions in other areas, highlighting the system's delicate balance and complex feedback mechanisms.

2.6 FINALLY, IT GETS BETTER

The food industry focuses on consumption without regard to health and illness prevention, while the health sector often overlooks the crucial role of diet in our well-being.

I spent some time in the last section talking about the impact of the medication's side effects on our body so let me refresh your memory about my journey until now. A few years after I started taking daily PPI medication the health problems started to develop. The chronologic list of the events is as follows:

- In 2009, I began taking a daily dose of PPI medication following a Barrett's esophagus diagnosis.
- By 2013, I had developed a vitamin B12 deficiency due to my body's inability to properly absorb the vitamin from food.
- The years between 2013 and 2020 were marked by severe abdominal pain, diarrhea, constipation, cramps, dizziness, and brain fog. My abdominal pain was so intense that I was afraid to go to the toilet by myself, scared that I would faint and hit my head in the fall.
- In the period between 2009 and 2016 despite regular endoscopies showing no alarming signs and no confirmation of Barrett's esophagus, my GI doctor continued prescribing PPIs.
- In 2016, I was diagnosed with Hashimoto's, an autoimmune disease. Seeking second and third opinions that year, despite my GI doctor insisting to take 2 doses of 40 mg PPIs per day, I was advised to stop taking PPIs as they weren't necessary for my GI issues.
- In 2016 I began the challenging process of transitioning from PPIs to H2-blockers, which took nearly half a year due to acid reflux rebound. This was also the year when I changed my GI doctor.
- A 2019 endoscopy revealed gastritis, yet the recommendation

was to keep taking H2-blockers medication.

- In October of 2020, due to bloating and abdominal pain another endoscopy indicated chronic gastritis, leading to a new prescription of PPIs.

Seven years of PPI medication and four years of H2-blocker medication later, I was now in the third quarter of 2020, with worse symptoms than when I started taking PPIs in 2009, with vitamin deficiencies and with at least one autoimmune disease developed. And the irony of it all is that I have been put on acid-blocking medication again, so back to how it all began and with worse symptoms than when it started.

I felt completely lost, with no one to turn to to explain why my body is failing me. Scared, frustrated and discouraged I decided that I wanted answers before following yet another medication treatment. I needed to take control over my health treatment, I needed to make sure that whoever was the medical professional that I was consulting, he/she does not follow blindly some set-in-stone procedures but is open-minded, up-to-date with latest developments in their specialty and willing to go few steps sideways from the procedures and treatment imposed by the medical community and to understand the root cause of my health issues.

I had a lot of questions and the only answer I got until now was "you have too much stomach acid":

- Why is my stomach irritated if I take powerful antacid medication?
- Does gastritis mean I have too much stomach acid or not enough?
- What is the root cause of my stomach being irritated?
- Is this irritation because I phased off the PPIs and therefore, by not having a strong medication to stop it my stomach is it secreting even more acid than before taking PPIs?
- But what about the H2-blocker medication, why does it not help to reduce the stomach acid if the acid is the issue? I still kept taking H2-blockers which lower the stomach acid so how much acid do I have that is causing the stomach lining to get inflamed?

- And if it is the too much acid that is the issue, why is my stomach secreting so much of it?

In summary, what is the root cause of my ailment? I needed to stop treating the symptom and start understanding and treating the cause.

It's noteworthy to mention that my journey with strong antacid medication began in 2009, prescribed by a GI doctor, despite not experiencing typical GERD symptoms such as discomfort after eating or while lying down. My sole symptom was an intense, debilitating pain in the upper stomach area, occurring three to four times a year. As I continued to take antacids at all other GI doctors' orders I started to develop symptoms of bloating, abdominal pain, dizziness, weakness, brain fog, fatigue, and hair loss. Every time I brought up my concerns that all these symptoms might be the result of the PPI's side effects, I have been dismissed, labeled as imagining things and prescribed antidepressants. Unfortunately, this is not only my story, but the one of other people that take long-term prescriptions for antacid medication. Being in touch with people that have autoimmune diseases I have discovered a pattern of behavior in our medical system: most of the patients feel dismissed, frustrated and helpless. Our concerns are not taken seriously, and we are ignored which makes some of us turn to various social media groups to find advice, similar experiences and get potential solutions. This is what I also did a few weeks later and it literally helped me much more in understanding the next steps I need to take to find a solution to my problems.

Worried that another regimen of strong PPI pills will increase my symptoms and might damage my already weakened body even more I asked the GI's registered nurse the question that was bugging me for some time now: "why do I have stomach irritated by acid if I do take one form or another of antacid?". The answer was "We don't know, but if you want, we can do some blood tests to get more insight".

WHAT???

There are tests that we can do to better understand the root cause, but I am put instead on PPIs just to calm down the symptom?

It was deeply troubling to observe the prevalent trend in healthcare where quick fixes in the form of prescription drugs, particularly Proton Pump Inhibitors (PPIs), are favored over comprehensive diagnostic efforts. This approach often overlooks the root causes of health issues, focusing instead on temporarily alleviating symptoms. This method, regrettably, leads to a cycle of dependency on medications that may bring a host of additional side effects.

This issue is a cause for concern not only for patients but also within the medical community. In my interactions, I've found that a significant number of healthcare professionals share this sense of frustration. They too are disillusioned with a system that seems to prioritize medication over more holistic healing methods. There's a palpable sense of dissatisfaction with the current medical practices that quickly resort to prescribing medication, which might offer immediate relief but fails to address the underlying health problems comprehensively.

On the flip side, there is also a challenge that healthcare providers face with patients who are resistant to making essential lifestyle changes. These patients often prefer the simplicity and immediacy of taking a pill to alleviate their symptoms, rather than committing to the more challenging path of lifestyle and dietary modifications. However, this preference for a quick pharmacological fix might stem from a lack of proper education and understanding. Many patients aren't sufficiently informed about the long-term consequences of relying on medications or the potential benefits that come with healthier lifestyle choices.

Moreover, this issue of inadequate knowledge isn't confined to patients alone. It appears that many medical professionals themselves might not be fully aware or convinced of the effectiveness of natural, non-pharmacological approaches to health. This gap in understanding and education extends throughout the healthcare system, affecting both the prescribers and the receivers of medical care. As a result, we find ourselves in a healthcare paradigm that often misses the opportunity for genuine healing and instead becomes trapped in a cycle of symptom management and medication dependence.

I do think that we need to introduce as early as elementary school classes on what a healthy diet is, methods to cope with stress, how to detox our lifestyle from all the chemicals in food, cleaning products, cosmetics and so on. This approach will foster a society more attuned to preventive healthcare. Beginning in elementary school, children can learn the fundamentals of a healthy diet, exploring the types of foods that nourish the body and contribute to overall well-being. Such education would not just cover the types of food to eat but also highlight the importance of balanced nutrition, the dangers of processed foods, and the benefits of whole, natural foods.

In addition to dietary education, these classes could incorporate lessons on managing stress. This aspect is crucial, as stress is a significant factor that affects health. Techniques like mindfulness, meditation, and simple breathing exercises could be taught to help students learn how to cope with stress from a young age. This knowledge would equip them with tools to manage their mental health as they grow older.

Furthermore, expanding the curriculum to include information about the chemicals found in everyday products, like cleaning agents and cosmetics, is equally important. Students can be educated about the potential health risks associated with certain chemicals and learn about safer alternatives. This knowledge would encourage them to make more informed choices about the products they use in their daily lives.

Carrying this education into secondary schools would allow for a deeper understanding and practical application of these concepts. As students mature, the curriculum can be expanded to cover more complex topics such as the long-term impacts of lifestyle choices on health, the importance of physical activity, and advanced nutritional concepts.

Additionally, it is crucial for medical education to incorporate comprehensive nutrition and lifestyle medicine courses. Medical professionals are often the first point of contact for individuals seeking health advice, and their guidance can significantly influence patient behaviors and outcomes. Therefore, equipping medical students with extensive knowledge about the role of diet, lifestyle, and environmental factors in health and disease prevention is essential. This shift in focus could help transform the healthcare system from one that often reacts to illnesses to one that proactively works to prevent them.

By starting health education early and continuing it through higher education, especially in medical schools, we can create a more health-conscious society. This approach has the potential to reduce the prevalence of lifestyle-related diseases and move towards a healthcare system that prioritizes prevention and holistic well-being.

I have digressed a little so let me go back on explaining what I did to regain my mental and physical health, in other words, my overall wellbeing. Let's be clear on one thing: once you acquire an autoimmune disease you cannot completely cure it but you can stop its progression and control the symptoms.

It was October of 2020, and my health is going from bad to worse without having any idea what I need to do to get better. The conventional medicine doctors were dismissing my concerns and they made me feel that I am complaining for no good reason. The GI's RN, at my insistence, ordered some blood tests and SURPRISE! My Antiparietal Cell Antibody test result was flagged as High, twice the value of the maximum accepted limit. You would expect to receive a phone call from your provider and explain the result, eventually change the course of the treatment, if necessary, right? WRONG! I did not receive any phone call. When I called, the answer was to continue the treatment given by my GI doctor, that is antacid medication.

Throughout my life, I've always sought to maintain control over my actions and life's direction. I've valued understanding my position, goals, and options, and crafting strategic plans to achieve my objectives. In retrospect, it puzzles me why I once relinquished total control of my health to a single doctor, rather than proactively seeking knowledge in this critical area. Today, given the vast resources available online and through social media, there's hardly any excuse for us as patients not to be well-informed. It's crucial that we advocate for ourselves and have the confidence to seek new medical opinions when we feel undervalued or misunderstood by healthcare professionals.

So, I needed to educate myself. I had no idea what having higher than the maximum accepted value for the Antiparietal Cell Antibody meant. I started small with a simple online search. This led to the discovery that my body's antibodies were attacking my stomach's Parietal Cells. What does this mean? Other online searches and logical deductions led me to realize that the destruction of these cells means reduced effectiveness in producing hydrochloric acid (HCl), contradicting my doctor's assumption of excessive stomach acid based on my stomach lining's irritation seen during endoscopy. From one logical thinking to another, from one discovery to another I concluded that I might have developed Autoimmune Gastritis (AIG). The treatment for this condition is NOT PPIs, nor H2-blockers. Since the stomach does not secrete enough HCl the prescription should be TAKING HCl in a pill form to help with the digestion to break down food and to act, also, as a natural defense mechanism against harmful pathogens, such as bacteria and viruses.

Another interesting discovery I made was that when Parietal Cells are impaired and unable to secrete hydrochloric acid (HCl), they also fail to produce Intrinsic Factor. This protein is critical for the absorption of vitamin B12. Reflecting on my experience from 2013, when blood tests indicated my B12 levels were barely within the acceptable range, the prescribed solution was B12 injections. However, this approach only addressed the symptom (B12 deficiency) without investigating the underlying cause — the probable lack of Intrinsic Factor due to impaired Parietal Cells. Both my family doctor and GI specialist missed an opportunity to delve deeper into the root cause of my B12 absorption issue. Ideally, medical investigations should aim to identify and treat the primary cause, rather than just managing the symptoms.

In cases like Autoimmune Gastritis, where the body's production of stomach acid is compromised, the standard treatments involving Proton Pump Inhibitors (PPIs) and H2-blockers is not suitable. Instead, an alternative treatment approach is the supplementation of hydrochloric acid (HCl) in pill form. This method compensates for the reduced acid production, aiding in the digestive process, facilitating the breakdown of food, and acting as a natural barrier against harmful pathogens. Such an approach targets the root cause of the condition — insufficient stomach acid production — rather than merely addressing its symptoms.

After a better understanding of the reason for having the stomach wall irritated, I needed to understand what the root cause and the treatment plan indicated by the conventional medicine were. Another online research showed that the root cause of autoimmune gastritis is not entirely clear, but it is believed to be a combination of genetic and environmental factors, one of them being other autoimmune conditions. People with other autoimmune conditions, such as type 1 diabetes, Hashimoto's thyroiditis, or celiac disease, may be at increased risk of developing autoimmune gastritis.

Now I started to have a common denominator that was bringing a little more light into the maze of separate diagnostics I got labeled with over the years: vitamin B12 deficiency in 2013, Hashimoto's in 2016 and chronic gastritis in 2020 (not defined as Autoimmune gastritis by my GI yet): autoimmune system went rogue and started to fight against parts of my body.

The treatment for autoimmune atrophic gastritis that is recommended by the conventional medicine is B12 injections and iron infusions. In case the endoscopy shows the formation of small neuroendocrine tumors, the GI doctor can remove them during the procedure with no risk since these tumors are usually non-cancerous. The treatment for the same disease recommended by Integrative medicine doctors is more comprehensive. In addition to vitamin B12, based on results from different tests that are not performed by conventional medicine yet, the treatment might involve other vitamins and minerals (if there is any deficiency in your body), an elimination diet that takes out different inflammatory items (remember that an autoimmune disease develops as a results of a chronic inflammation), stress management and other holistic approaches.

But why am I developing autoimmune diseases? I don't have any genetic predisposition to autoimmune diseases so what was the reason for my autoimmune system to mistakenly attack my own cells? These perplexing questions led me down various online research paths, yet a satisfactory answer eluded me.

Feeling powerless and hopeless one day I confided in my son about my debilitating symptoms and my waning hope in conventional medical solutions. It was through this act of sharing and his subsequent discussions with his friends that I was introduced to a book on autoimmune diseases. This marked a turning point in my journey towards recovery.

The insights gained from this book, combined with my own research, opened new avenues for understanding and managing my health. This experience underscored the power of sharing our struggles and seeking knowledge beyond traditional sources, although I recognize the importance of balancing this with professional medical guidance. I'm immensely grateful for this pivotal moment, sparked by a conversation with my son, which steered me toward a path of proactive health management.

In my quest to pinpoint an accurate diagnosis, I embraced the role of a meticulous investigator. Beyond the surface-level symptoms, I delved into a diverse array of medical studies and resources. This exploration spanned topics from the side effects of Proton Pump Inhibitors (PPIs) to the intricacies of autoimmune diseases like Hashimoto's. I also investigated how stress, our dietary choices, and environmental factors contribute to both the emergence and healing of health issues. This journey into the depths of medical research wasn't just about finding answers; it was about taking an active, informed role in my health care. While I recognize the indispensable role of medical professionals in interpreting these findings, my foray into these studies was a crucial step in understanding the complex web of factors influencing my health.

I started to read a lot of books on autoimmune disease. There is a plethora of educational information for us as patients but most importantly for the medical practitioners. Over the past decade, remarkable strides have been made in understanding the crucial role of gut health in influencing both our physical and mental well-being. My reading journey not only enriched my knowledge but also shed light on the limitations and inaccuracies of the treatment I had been following. These insights helped me understand the vital connection between our digestive health and overall health, highlighting how imbalances in the gut can lead to a spectrum of issues, from mood disorders to severe physical ailments.

In addition to spending every free moment I had, day and mostly nights and weekends, reading medical studies and books as if my life depended on it (and it literally did), I started to search some Facebook groups that have as the main subject a certain illness. I realized soon that there are amazingly good, well managed groups that offer invaluable information. Autoimmune Atrophic Gastritis & Pernicious Anemia, Hashimoto's 411, AIP Diet Support Group, The Kidney Stone Prevention Diet are just some of them. Each is led by very knowledgeable admins and the files posted are a wealth of information on the specific subject. The members of these groups are very respectful and supportive.

In my journey through various online communities, I encountered a spectrum of experiences. Some groups, unfortunately, were marred by disrespectful interactions and seemed more focused on promoting specific medications rather than fostering a supportive environment for sharing up-to-date information and mutual help. Particularly in one group dedicated to Barrett's Esophagus, I observed a strong bias towards promoting PPIs as the sole treatment, often dismissing members' concerns about side effects like dizziness, joint pain, anemia, and vertigo. When evidence questioning the effectiveness of PPIs in managing Barrett's Esophagus was presented, the responses from the administrators were dismissive and sometimes impolite. This led me to leave those groups, choosing instead to continue my self-education within more constructive and open-minded online spaces.

The turning point in my educational journey was understanding the profound influence of diet on health. Throughout life, from childhood to adulthood, many of us unknowingly harm our bodies with our dietary choices. It wasn't until a pivotal moment that I acknowledged the need for a dietary overhaul to ensure not just a longer life, but one of better quality. Aside from a brief phase after moving to Canada, where I lost control over my eating habits, I believed I was eating reasonably well. My diet mostly consisted of moderate portions of meat (primarily chicken, turkey, and occasionally high-quality beef), a variety of vegetables, and weekly servings of seeds and legumes.

I started the AIP elimination diet at the beginning of December 2020, and I followed it until sometime in March 2021. Since then, I introduced some food items but I still prefer not to introduce some others at all and I will go into detail on my decisions in the next chapter.

In December 2020, I already read a lot about Hashimoto's, Pernicious Anemia and Autoimmune Gastritis and I started the AIP diet, but I still did not find any medical professional with whom I can talk about finding the root cause of my problems and not only giving me hard-medication to ease my symptoms. Reading Dr. Amy Myers' book, "The Autoimmune Solution", I realized that there is another type of doctors, the Functional Medicine doctors, that do treat exactly what I wanted: the root cause of the problem.

It's essential to recognize that everyone's body is unique, and what works for one person might not be effective for another. This individuality is why I was cautious about blindly following others' paths in terms of supplement use. I also do not recommend starting a certain treatment based only on what a book says or on the advice you receive from different emails or social media. I believe that treatment should be tailored to each individual, guided by concrete data from medical tests rather than anecdotal evidence or hearsay. This approach ensures that any treatment or supplement regimen I adopt is specifically suited to my body's needs and conditions, rather than a one-size-fits-all solution.

It's crucial to work with a doctor who not only adopts a holistic approach but also stays abreast of the latest medical discoveries. Medicine is a constantly evolving field with new research, treatments, and technologies emerging regularly. This combination of holistic and conventional medicine ensures a more comprehensive understanding of one's health that considers all aspects of an individual's life, including physical, emotional, social, and environmental factors.

After realizing the need for a Functional Medicine practitioner, I specifically sought an M.D. with a solid medical background, ideally a good internist and diagnostician. My research led me to Dr. Susan Blum, the founder of Blum Center for Health. However, I hesitated initially to book an appointment due to the substantial costs involved. Functional Medicine consultations are expensive, and as a new patient, the fees were particularly high. Moreover, the specialized tests recommended by these practitioners are typically not covered by insurance.

My hesitation was further compounded by the financial aspect. It felt overwhelming to commit such a significant amount of money, knowing that insurance wouldn't offset the costs. The turning point came when my husband pointed out my willingness to spend a similar amount on an eye surgery for our 15-year-old dog, yet I was reluctant to invest in my own health. This comparison puts things into perspective, underscoring the importance of prioritizing my well-being. His words resonated with me, leading me to finally decide to schedule an appointment with Dr. Blum.

Choosing Dr. Blum as my doctor proved to be one of the wisest decisions I've made. She embodies the qualities I sought in a physician: intelligence, a logical approach, and a strong emphasis on factual evidence. Dr. Blum's methodology is thorough and precise, focusing on identifying and addressing the underlying causes of health issues rather than merely alleviating symptoms. This approach aligns with my belief that symptoms naturally resolve when the root cause is effectively treated. I am deeply grateful for her expertise and care, and I sincerely believe that her intervention has been lifesaving for me.

2.6.1 LABORATORY TESTS

I believe it's crucial for individuals to understand that solely relying on blood tests may not always reveal thyroid disorders. Some results may appear normal, but they are not optimum. This leads me to think that there are likely many more people suffering the symptoms of thyroid conditions and are not officially diagnosed with this disease.

The first session with her was towards the end of January 2021 and it lasted around two hours. During this time, we went over my whole life, from when I was born until that present time, discussing all the main aspects of my life, the diseases, the stresses, the medication. In short, all my health life's history. At the end of that first session, I got prescription for several special tests:

1. **GI MAP** – also known as the Gastrointestinal Microbial Assay Plus, represents a significant advancement in the understanding and treatment of gastrointestinal health. Its comprehensive approach to analyzing the gut microbiome offers valuable insights, leading to more effective and personalized treatments for various gut-related health issues. As I mentioned previously, 70 to 80% of our immune system is in the gut therefore, a healthy gut is very important for the health of our physical body and our mind. This test is different from the one that is performed, albeit very rarely, by conventional medicine doctors and it is not covered by the insurance.

This test provides valuable information about the composition of the gut microbiota and detects the presence of various microorganisms, including bacteria, parasites, fungi, and viruses, allowing medical providers to assess overall balance of the gut microbiome and identify any potential imbalances or dysfunctions. The GI Map test uses advanced molecular techniques to identify and quantify specific genetic material from the microorganisms present in a stool sample and provides information about various markers such as:

- **Microbial pathogens:** identifies harmful microorganisms such as pathogenic bacteria (Salmonella, Campylobacter), parasites (Giardia, Cryptosporidium, Blastocystis hominis) and viruses (norovirus).
- **Opportunistic pathogens:** Recognizes microorganisms that can become problematic under certain conditions, such as Candida species, which may cause yeast overgrowth.
- **Normal flora:** Evaluates the levels of beneficial bacteria in the gut, like Bifidobacterium and Lactobacillus.
- **Inflammatory markers:** measures the presence of markers associated with inflammation in the gut (calprotectin).

Using the GI-Map test information the medical providers can have a better understanding of a potential root cause helping them in providing a more accurate diagnosis and offer a personalized treatment plan, including dietary and probiotic interventions to restore gut health and improve overall well-being. This test is very helpful in diagnosing several conditions like IBS, IBD, gut dysbiosis, abdominal pain, depression, brain fog amongst others.

One friend of mine expressed her concern that the tests prescribed by the functional medicine doctors are not peer-reviewed and therefore the procedure is not generally accepted by the medical community. It's worth noting though that the field of microbiome analysis and diagnostic tests is a relatively new and rapidly evolving area of research. Peer-reviewed studies often take time to be conducted, published, and subsequently reviewed by the scientific community. The lack of extensive peer-reviewed research at this time does not diminish the clinical potential of these tests but highlights the need for ongoing research and validation in this emerging field.

2. The **Metabolomix** test, offered by Genova Diagnostics, is a comprehensive urine test that evaluates various markers related to nutritional status and metabolism. This test is particularly insightful for individuals experiencing a range of symptoms, including:

- Mood disorders
- Growth issues
- Muscle weakness or pain
- Digestive issues like diarrhea or constipation
- Seizures
- Autism spectrum disorders
- Sensory impairments (visual or hearing problems)
- Chronic fatigue
- Persistent stress
- Inflammation
- Unexplained weight gain

By analyzing these markers, the Metabolomix test can provide valuable information about a person's nutritional needs, potential imbalances, and deficiencies. This insight is crucial in understanding how diet and nutrition impact overall health and well-being. For instance, it can reveal specific needs for vitamins, minerals, and amino acids, helping tailor dietary and supplement regimens to the unique requirements of each individual.

This personalized approach to nutrition and supplementation is particularly important because, like medications, supplements can have side effects, especially if taken in excess or without a clear need. Therefore, the Metabolomix test can guide individuals in making more informed choices about their health, ensuring they only take supplements that are beneficial for their specific health conditions, lifestyle, and stress levels. This not only promotes better health outcomes but also helps in avoiding unnecessary expenses on supplements that might not be necessary or could potentially be harmful.

A typical Metabolomix test includes the following information:

- **Nutrient Needs** (Antioxidants, B-Vitamins, Minerals) and Toxic Elements: This aspect of the test evaluates the levels of essential nutrients and potential toxic elements in the body, identifying nutritional deficiencies or exposures to harmful substances.

- **Amino Acids**: Amino acids are fundamental components of proteins. The Metabolomix test assesses potential imbalances in amino acids, providing insights into nutrient deficiencies or metabolic issues.
- **Organic Acids:** These are metabolic byproducts found in urine. Their analysis can offer valuable insights into nutrient metabolism, energy production, detoxification processes, gut health, and oxidative stress. It can help in understanding the efficiency of various metabolic pathways.
- **Essential and Metabolic Fatty Acids** (e.g., Omega-3 and Omega-6): This component assesses fat metabolism, indicating any imbalances or deficiencies in essential fatty acids. It's crucial for maintaining cellular function and overall health.
- **Oxidative Stress Markers:** These markers reveal cellular damage that may be caused by oxidative stress, which is an imbalance between free radicals (natural byproducts of metabolism) and the body's ability to counteract their harmful effects. Oxidative stress can be influenced by factors like:
- Environmental pollutants, toxins and radiation exposure
- Unhealthy diet and lifestyle choices
- Chronic stress
- Certain diseases such as diabetes, autoimmune diseases, and chronic inflammation

3.**DUTCH** test is a comprehensive hormone testing procedure that analyzes hormone metabolites in dried urine samples. The acronym stands for Dried Urine Test for Comprehensive Hormones, and it provides detailed insights into a person's hormonal balance and overall hormonal health. The test measures the following hormones and metabolites:

- **Estrogens Metabolism:** This aspect assesses estrogen levels and potential imbalances, which are crucial for understanding various health conditions, particularly in reproductive health.
- **Progesterone Levels**: The test measures its levels, offering insights into various reproductive and menstrual health issues.

- **Cortisol Levels:** Cortisol is a critical hormone affecting energy levels, stress response, and sleep patterns. This analysis helps in understanding stress-related disorders and adrenal health.
- **Melatonin Levels**: The test assesses melatonin levels, which can provide insights into sleep disorders and overall sleep health.
- **Hormone Metabolites**: The test also includes an analysis of hormone metabolites, providing detailed information on how the body processes and metabolizes hormones. This can be key in understanding hormonal imbalances and their potential impact on the body.

The DUTCH test is particularly useful for diagnosing and managing conditions such as adrenal fatigue, mood disorders, menstrual irregularities, and fertility issues.

4. **SIBO**, or Small Intestinal Bacterial Overgrowth, is diagnosed using a breath test that measures hydrogen and methane gasses. These gasses are byproducts of bacterial metabolism in the small intestine. The test is straightforward and non-invasive, aiding healthcare providers in accurately diagnosing SIBO and formulating effective treatment strategies to manage the bacterial overgrowth.

Under normal conditions, the small intestine contains fewer bacteria compared to the large intestine. However, when there is an unusual increase in the quantity or type of bacteria in the small intestine, a range of symptoms may occur, including:

- **Abdominal Pain:** This can vary in intensity from mild to severe.
- **Bloating:** Caused by excessive gas production from bacterial metabolism.
- **Diarrhea:** Occurs due to disruption in normal digestion.
- **Constipation:** Can be a result of slowed intestinal motility.
- **Belching or Flatulence:** Increased gas production leads to these symptoms.

- **Abdominal Cramps:** Inflammation and gas production can cause cramping.

- **Nutritional Deficiencies:** Bacterial activity can interfere with the absorption of vitamins and minerals.

- **Fatigue and Weakness:** Stem from nutrient malabsorption and ongoing inflammation.

- **Weight Loss, Heartburn, Acid Reflux, Nausea, Joint Pain:** These are additional symptoms that may accompany SIBO.

SIBO can significantly disturb the equilibrium of the gut microbiota, highlighting the importance of its accurate diagnosis and thorough treatment. It's a condition that necessitates careful medical attention due to its potential to cause widespread disturbances in gastrointestinal and overall health.

5. **Blood tests** – In addition to the normal blood tests that any conventional medicine doctor is prescribing, based on the symptom that one person is displaying there are other special tests that need to be performed. Here are some of the tests I did based on my symptoms that I explained in previous chapters:

    - **Complete Blood Count (CBC)** – shows if there is any abnormality in the blood cells counts (red blood cells, white blood cells, platelets).

    - **Antinuclear Antibodies (ANA)** – it detects the presence of antibodies that target the cell nucleus components. It can indicate several autoimmune diseases such as systemic lupus erythematosus (SLE), Sjogren syndrome, forms of arthritis.

    - **Parietal cell antibodies (PCA)** – detects the autoantibodies that target the stomach parietal cells. As discussed in detail previously, they are specialized to produce hydrochloric acid and intrinsic factor. The presence of parietal cell antibodies is associated with diseases like Autoimmune Gastritis which leads to impaired digestion and B12 deficiency and Pernicious Anemia which is a type of anemia characterized by vitamin B12 deficiency.

- **Comprehensive Metabolic Panel (CMP)** – assesses the health of liver, kidney, pancreas and evaluates the electrolyte balance and blood sugar levels. This test is part of a yearly routine health screening.
- **Thyroid Function Tests** - assess the thyroid functionality and to detect specific thyroid antibodies:
- **Thyroid-Stimulating Hormone (THS)** levels are an indication of an underactive thyroid (hypothyroidism if THS levels are elevated) or an overactive thyroid (hyperthyroidism if the THS levels are low).
- **Thyroid Peroxidase Antibodies (TPOAb)** is associated with Hashimoto's thyroiditis when levels are elevated.
- **Thyroglobulin Antibodies (TgAb)** is also associated with Hashimoto's thyroiditis and at the same time with Grave's disease.
- **Free Thyroxine (FT4)** and **Free Triiodothyronine (FT3)** measure the levels of FT4 and FT3 respectively.
- **Nutrients for Thyroid Function:** nutrients needed for an optimal thyroid function such as: Iron/Ferritin, Vitamin D, Vitamin A, Homocysteine, Selenium, Zinc, Magnesium.
- **DHEA Sulfate** – provides information about the overall function of the adrenal glands and it is also used in evaluating androgen production, especially in polycystic ovary syndrome (PCOS).
- **High-Sensitivity C-Reactive protein (HS CRP)** test measures a protein produced by the liver in response to inflammation in the body. It is associated with the risk of developing a cardiovascular disease.

Based on the symptoms a person is exhibiting some other tests might be ordered:

- **Erythrocyte Sedimentation Rate (ESR)** – same as the CRP test, high ESR levels give indication of the presence of an inflammatory autoimmune disease.

- **Rheumatoid Factor (RF)** is normally used to diagnose rheumatoid arthritis.

- **Anti-SSA (Ro) and Anti-SSB (La)** Antibodies is performed if Sjorgren's syndrome is suspected, affecting the tear and salivary glands.

- **Anti-Tissue Transglutaminase (anti-tTG)** Antibodies and Total IgA are two tests used for diagnosing celiac disease which is an autoimmune condition triggered by the ingestion of gluten.

- **Anti-Smooth Muscle Antibodies (ASMA)** and Liver Function tests help to evaluate autoimmune hepatitis and liver function in general.

- **Anti-Double-Stranded DNA (anti-dsDNA)** antibodies are specific to validate the diagnosis of systemic lupus erythematosus.

In the realm of healthcare, especially when dealing with chronic and complex health conditions, the role of a Functional Medicine Doctor becomes pivotal.

My journey with conventional medicine left several of my health issues unaddressed. For example, despite persistent and varied gastrointestinal symptoms, conventional doctors did not suggest a stool test. Had such a test been performed earlier, it could have identified the presence of Blastocystis hominis. This parasite is known to cause significant gastrointestinal issues and inflammation, and its detection could have radically changed my treatment plan and possibly alleviated many of my symptoms.

Similarly, no conventional medicine doctor has prescribed any test to evaluate my body's hormonal health. Had they done it they would have found out I had adrenal fatigue with an imbalance of cortisone and cortisol which gave me a complete lack of energy in the morning and during the day and an overactive state as the evening started. I had problems getting asleep and staying asleep. Since I discovered the existence of autoimmune diseases in addition to reading a lot of books on this subject, I also started to listen to diverse podcasts to help me better understand how to treat them. One day, I listened to a conventional medicine doctor who was denying the existence of adrenal fatigue. In her opinion, this was an invention, more of a scam of the functional medicine field with the only purpose of making money when prescribing the specialty tests. I might have agreed with her had I not been diagnosed and treated for adrenal fatigue based on the data from the above tests. The supplements (not hard medication) prescribed by my functional medicine doctor for a limited period of time helped me rebalance the hormones and get the quality sleep I needed to help my body get to its optimal functions. The effectiveness of this approach was evident in the significant improvement in my overall well-being. After a certain period, once my hormonal balance was restored, I was able to discontinue the supplements. For the past year and a half, I have maintained excellent health, a testament to the success of the treatment.

No conventional medicine doctor was curious to do tests to better assess the health of my thyroid gland before prescribing hard medication after a minimum of blood tests. Had they done that they might have seen that some of the vitamin and mineral levels in my blood were not normal and maybe only by bringing them to optimal levels I might have been spared of taking life-long, daily medication.

No conventional medicine doctor tried to understand the minerals and vitamins deficiencies in my body. Had they done it they would have found out that only by stopping the PPIs and prescribing supplements to replenish my cells with them would have given me the energy to do the day-to-day activities.

No conventional medicine doctor added all my symptoms together and looked at me as a whole. Each doctor saw me through the eyes of his/her specialty disregarding the symptoms that did not fit in the box of their field. Had they done that, I might have saved years of suffering, hundreds of thousands of dollars spent on tests, endoscopies and other procedures and surely, I would not have written this book.

Furthermore, no conventional medicine doctor even questioned me about my diet, my stress levels, and my exercise routine. Had they done that they would have found out that my stress levels were high, and my diet was not appropriate for the new symptoms I experienced. But for them to even think about diet and lifestyle, the doctors would have to have in the curriculum of medical school these subjects and study them in more detail than what the school offers today.

Functional medicine, in my case, provided a solution that conventional approaches had overlooked or dismissed over and over again.

My story is a reminder of the diverse approaches in medicine and the need for an open-minded yet critical evaluation of all available treatment options. We need a healthcare system that embraces a comprehensive approach, combining the strengths of both conventional and functional medicine to offer the best possible care tailored to individual needs.

The absence of a holistic approach in conventional medicine often leads to fragmented care, where symptoms are treated in isolation, and the underlying causes remain unexplored. This is where Functional Medicine doctors play a crucial role. They often use a wide array of diagnostic tools, including comprehensive blood tests, stool analysis, hormone testing, and more, to build a detailed picture of a patient's health.

By examining factors like dietary habits, environmental exposures, genetic predisposition, and lifestyle choices, a Functional Medicine practitioner can develop a personalized treatment plan. This plan often includes dietary changes, lifestyle modifications, and supplements targeted to address specific deficiencies or imbalances.

My experience highlighted the importance of advocating for one's health and seeking out practitioners willing to look beyond standard protocols. It is essential for patients to find doctors who are partners in their health journey, willing to listen, investigate deeply, and consider all aspects of their health. This collaborative approach is often more effective in treating chronic conditions and improving overall well-being.

Autoimmune diseases are difficult to identify, and many patients suffer for years without a medical diagnosis. But this is mainly due to the lack of testing either because the doctor refuses to prescribe (a lot of patients are complaining about this) or because the insurance refuses to approve the test.

If I can simplify, every cell in our body regenerates every seven years. In this process, the antibodies we produce get rid of the old and damaged cells to make room for new cells. Normally, we have antibodies for every part of our body and are in normal ranges but when we have elevated antibodies our own self kills off more cells than we are making, and this is how the damage is done and the autoimmune diseases start. Whether it has produced symptoms or not depends on how long this process has been going on and how much tissue we have lost because of the elevated antibodies. Detection of predictive biomarkers in the early stages of autoimmune disorders can be used to identify, halt, and even reverse autoimmune diseases. Latest studies on predictive autoimmunity show that if you have any elevated antibodies to erythematosus lupus, the positive predictive value that you are getting lupus is 94 to 100% within seven to ten years, elevated scleroderma antibodies show a positive predictive value of 100% within 11 years, for Rheumatoid arthritis the value is 52 to 97% within 14 years, for Crohn's disease if you have ASCA antibodies, the positive predictive value is 100% in three years. For many of the autoimmune diseases we know now what the positive predictive value is in order to be officially diagnosed with this disease and about how long before you are going to feel it with all its symptoms unless you detect it early and you take steps to stop it and even reverse it.

All this shows that the latest discoveries give us the means to detect in very early stages, long before we feel any symptom, the development of an autoimmune disease, if only the biomarkers tests would be performed. The sad part of it all is that even when the symptoms are there, and we are doubled down in pain, the diagnosis, and the treatment we get are based on guessing instead of based on data and with the complexity of our system this could easily lead to misdiagnosis and years of pain and medical expenses.

Early detection and intervention can be crucial in managing and potentially reversing the course of autoimmune diseases. Understanding the risk factors and early signs, and taking proactive steps in consultation with healthcare professionals, can significantly alter the disease trajectory.

Before going forward to explain the treatment I got and how I started to feel better I would like to talk briefly about the lab results and their ranges of acceptance.

Normally, when you do a blood test or any type of test you feel relieved when the results fall within the reference range, even if the result is close to the minimum or the maximum side of the range. But are we correct assuming we are not sick in this case? Most doctors do not prescribe any treatment if the test result is close to the limits of the range despite the fact that you exhibit symptoms of deficiency. I heard a lot of women complaining that their doctor does not prescribe vitamin B12 injections even though their vitamin B12 serum was in the low two hundreds (reference range: 200-1100 pg/mL) and they presented symptoms such as fatigue and lack of energy, general weakness, dizziness and some experienced even "pins and needles" sensation in the hands and feet.

So, how are the reference ranges established and why do they vary from one laboratory to another?

Reference ranges for the lab tests are typically established statistically, collecting samples from a large number of individuals recruited to represent the target population.

The desired samples are collected (blood, urine, saliva, and others) and the tests are performed measuring the different parameters of interest. The results are then analyzed statistically establishing the mean (average), the standard deviation and the percentiles which will become the basis for the reference ranges. The lower and upper limits of the range are usually defined as the 2.5th and 97.5th percentiles respectively.

Reference ranges can vary between different laboratories based on their internal procedure, the individuals who represent the target population and the lab instrumentation.

In theory, these individuals who represent the target population are screened to ensure they are healthy, however, since a lot of chronic diseases are difficult to diagnose in early stages of the disease when the symptoms do not manifest yet, and since a lot of discoveries on autoimmunity, gut health and genetics are not older than 10 – 15 years, there is a strong possibility that some of the individuals chosen to represent the target population and considered "healthy" might be in fact be in the early stages of a chronic condition. Moreover, the normal screening tests do not show an overall picture of the health of an individual.

That is why the reference ranges should not be taken as a diagnostic cutoff. They should be interpreted in the context of each individual's clinical symptoms and taking into consideration the patient's health history, current lifestyle (diet, stress level, medication), age, gender, and sometimes other demographic characteristics. Depending on the test, if in general it is desirable to have your test result in the middle of the reference range, for some conditions it is better to have it towards the higher side of the range.

If you think of all these variables one must stop to consider that being a doctor is not an easy task: a doctor should have the curiosity of a child to understand all the symptoms and the health history of the patient and to do follow ups to see if the treatment is successful; should have the empathy needed to actively listen and to understand the patient's emotions and pains, the logic and mindset of a detective to put everything together, to look at the patient as a whole and not as an organ learned in school and come up with a logical diagnosis and the treatment for the root cause and not for the symptoms. For all this to happen, the medical school has to offer a better training (including the impact of the diet and the stress on the mental and physical body, including the interaction of all our organs and systems on the overall health), the doctors should not be pressed by time to see the maximum number of patients within an hour timeframe and the insurance companies should let the doctors do their job instead of limiting their options.

2.6.2 PERSONALIZED TREATMENT

Individualized care in medicine should prioritize the needs and well-being of the patient over the financial or operational efficiencies of the healthcare system.

I consider myself very lucky that I learned, albeit later than I would have liked, about functional medicine and that I decided to follow up my health treatment with a trained doctor. But before I did that, I read books, medical studies and listened to podcasts related to autoimmune diseases in general, and in particular about gastritis, Hashimoto's, and thyroid gland in general, so I was generally quite well educated in the complications of an autoimmune disease.

A month before having my first appointment with Dr. Blum I completely eliminated the gluten, dairy, legumes, and sugar from my alimentation, and I started the AIP diet. Reading about the benefits of meditation and controlled breathing on the stress management I scheduled daily time for such activities. I read about the importance of vitamins (B12, D, C), minerals (Mg, Fe) on the overall health of the thyroid gland so I was not surprised when the doctor ordered the tests I just talked about.

My first appointment lasted two hours at the end of which I was left with prescriptions for different special tests, listed previously, and with the suggestion to meet the Center's dictitian. The next session was a couple of months later, after all the test results were available.

Based on my test results I had the first personalized treatment plan:

- **Gut health** – the GI MAP stool test showed low abundance in good bacteria, high occurrence of Blastocystis hominis parasite and low IgA (Immunoglobulin A). IgA is a type of antibody that plays an important role in the immune system's defense by recognizing and neutralizing viruses, bacteria, and other pathogens. It maintains a healthy balance of microorganisms in the gut.

The first priority was to treat the parasite with a 10-day treatment. At the same time, I was put on **Saccharomyces Boulardii**, a beneficial yeast used as a dietary supplement to support gastrointestinal health. S. Boulardii is a probiotic that has been studied and used in the management of various gastrointestinal conditions such as traveler's diarrhea, IBS and IBD.

Once I finished the parasite treatment, I started to take **oil of oregano** capsules. It has a long history of use in traditional medicine, and it is believed to have antibacterial, antiviral, and antifungal effects. It is also believed to have antimicrobial effects against certain harmful bacteria that can cause digestive problems and to boost the immune health, improving the defenses against infections.

To improve the IgA, in addition to S. Boulardii I started to take **SBI** (Serum-derived Bovine Immunoglobulin) powder twice daily. SBI powder is thought to maintain the integrity of the intestinal lining and to support the barrier function of the gut. It is recommended for leaky gut syndrome, IBS, IBD and food sensitivities. The immunoglobulins it contains provide additional antibodies that might promote a diverse and healthy balanced gut microbiome.

- **Hormones, sleep, and fatigue** – the DUTCH test revealed that my adrenals are low. My cortisol levels were at the lower limit at the waking moment, dropping in the morning below the lowest range limit and increasing towards the highest range limit in the evening. This explains the energy I had before going to bed and the fatigue I was experiencing during the morning and the rest of the day.

    My adrenals were worn out. The adrenal glands, located on top of each kidney, produce and release various hormones like cortisol, aldosterone, adrenaline (epinephrine) and noradrenaline (norepinephrine). Cortisol is involved in regulating stress response, metabolism, immune function, blood pressure and inflammation. Adrenaline and noradrenaline are involved in the "fight or flight" response and preparing the body to mobilize stored energy for the coming stress or danger.

Cortisol levels vary throughout the day, being typically highest in the morning and gradually decreasing during the day with the lowest level reached before going to bed. Proper regulation of cortisol is essential for the immune function of the body, for the sleep-wake cycle and for the stress response.

My poor stress management knowledge combined with being continuously in a "fight or flight" state since I immigrated 27 years ago, have worn out my adrenal glands and the hormone levels did not follow the natural, healthy path anymore.

To treat the low adrenals, I had to implement a plan to improve my lifestyle and my stress management skills. I continued daily meditation that I started a couple of months before, I increased the time I spent outside, and I tried to be mindful and enjoy every moment I spent in nature. The breathing exercises helped me to control my reaction in the stressful moments and changing my mindset has helped me realize what is really important in my life and stop reacting to what is less important.

In addition to these lifestyle changes, I started to take a couple of herbal supplements: **Adrenal support** and Cortisol manager. The doctor also added **DHEA** since the blood tests showed low levels which is common with adrenal fatigue.

- **Stomach health and heartburn** – First of all I had to stop taking any antacid medication, so I stopped the H2-blockers.

  To control the heartburn, I started to take DGL (deglycyrrhizinated licorice) chewable tablets. DGL is known for soothing effects on the digestive system and to alleviate symptoms of heartburn by promoting a healthy mucus lining in the stomach and esophagus, providing thus a protective barrier against the stomach acid. It is believed that the flavonoids found in licorice which have antioxidant and anti-inflammatory properties may be responsible for the potential health benefits of DGL.

Another method I used to control the heartburn was taking Heartburn Tx powder around two hours after lunch and dinner at the beginning and later on only after dinner. The combination of ingredients (Aloe Vera, Zinc, L-Glutamine, N-Acetyl-Glucosamine, DGL) soothe the GI tract and maintain the integrity of the mucosal lining.

Herbal teas are other supplements I used, such as slippery elm and marshmallow root, beneficial for gut health and for promoting a healthy esophagus and stomach lining, while chamomile and linden teas were helpful in helping me relax. Milk thistle and dandelion root herbal teas helped me restore the good function of my liver.

- **Vitamins and mineral deficiencies** – Blood and Metabolomix test results indicated the need for taking some supplements to compensate for my body's inability to assimilate those from my diet. Vitamin B12, D, and B2 were some of them so I was prescribed a B complex and a Multivitamin to take daily in addition to sublingual B12 (methylcobalamin) and a vitamin D3 pill that I was also taking daily. There is a lot of discussion about taking B12 liquid sublingual instead of injections. The belief is that for a person who has problems assimilating due to damaged parietal cells and therefore to lack of intrinsic factor any other type of oral vitamin B12 other than injections will not be assimilated to the cell level. I believe that this might vary from person to person. The liquid sublingual B12 is assimilated into the bloodstream through the mucous membranes located under our tongue. They are more permeable than other areas of the oral cavity. This option is non-invasive and can be easily administered at home compared with injecting the B12. While effective, the absorption rate can vary depending on individual factors like the health of mucous membranes and consistency in administration. Both methods are effective for supplementing B12, but the choice between sublingual administration and injections depends on the severity of the deficiency, the underlying cause of the deficiency, patient preference, and how the body responds to each form of supplementation. For some, sublingual B12 is sufficient and more convenient, while others may require the more immediate and assured absorption provided by injections. Regardless of the method of supplementing with B12 some blood tests can give a good indication to evaluate B12 at cellular level:

- o **Methylmalonic Acid (MMA):** High levels of MMA in the blood or urine can indicate B12 deficiency at the cellular level. Vitamin B12 is necessary for converting MMA to succinic acid, so elevated MMA suggests that this conversion isn't happening efficiently due to inadequate B12.

- o **Homocysteine:** This is an amino acid in the blood that requires B12 (as well as folate and Vitamin B6) for its metabolism. Elevated homocysteine levels can indicate a deficiency in one or more of these nutrients, including B12. However, high homocysteine can also be influenced by other factors, such as kidney disease and genetic predispositions.

- o **Holotranscobalamin (Holotc or Active B12 Test):** Holotranscobalamin is a test that measures the amount of vitamin B12 attached to transcobalamin, which is the form of B12 that is readily available for cellular uptake. This can be a more direct measure of the B12 that is actually usable by the body's cells.

- o Complete Blood Count (CBC): While not a direct measure of B12 at the cellular level, a CBC can provide indirect indications. For example, macrocytic anemia (enlarged red blood cells) is a common sign of B12 deficiency, although it can have other causes as well.

It's important to note that interpreting these tests can be complex and should be done by a healthcare professional. Often, a combination of these tests, along with a review of symptoms and medical history, is used to get a more accurate picture of an individual's B12 status. Each test has its own limitations and might be influenced by factors other than B12

- **Liver enzymes** – my liver enzymes (ALT, AST) came back elevated, so the doctor added some liver protection supplements to my battery of supplements I had to take daily. **Liver Protect** supplement contains milk thistle, which is known for antioxidant and anti-inflammatory effect, dandelion root traditionally used to stimulate bile production and to eliminate toxins from the liver, artichoke extract thought to promote bile production helping with the digestion and absorption of fats and N-acetylcysteine (NAC) which helps glutathione production, an important antioxidant and detoxifier. Once my liver enzymes got to acceptable levels, I discontinued using these supplements and the levels remained stable since then.

- **Hashimoto's and autoimmunity** - the decision was to continue taking Levothyroxine, alternating between 50mg and 75mg, since the thyroid antibodies (TPO Ab and Tg Ab) were at a steady level.

- **The lifestyle** – my main focus was to manage how I perceive and how I react to stress and to improve my sleeping pattern. Writing down a "to do" list for the next day, keeping a journal, taking a walk before going to bed, and in the morning after waking up, avoiding any electronics at least one hour before going to bed, exposing your eyes to the day light within 15 to 30 minutes after waking up to help your circadian rhythm, exercise, are only some of the techniques I used to get my body back on a healthy path.

- **The diet** – Three months after embarking on my AIP diet journey, I reached a pivotal moment where I felt ready to reintroduce certain foods back into my diet. This step was crucial, not only to diversify my meals but also to ensure I was benefiting from a broader spectrum of nutrients essential for my health.

To this day, I maintain a strict avoidance of gluten, dairy, sugar, soy, corn, and nightshades. These were the culprits I identified early on as triggers for my autoimmune symptoms, and steering clear of them has been instrumental in my wellbeing. However, I've welcomed legumes back into my diet once or twice per week.

Eating out, which once seemed daunting, is now something I approach with confidence. I've learned to navigate menus and communicate my dietary needs to restaurant staff, ensuring that I can enjoy a meal out without compromising my health.

Perhaps one of the most enjoyable aspects of this journey has been developing my personalized recipes. I've experimented with various ingredients that align with the AIP guidelines and suit my palate. I've discovered that dietary restrictions don't necessarily mean sacrificing flavor or pleasure in eating. For instance, I've mastered the art of creating desserts that are both delicious and compliant with my dietary needs. I use natural sweeteners like honey, maple syrup, and coconut sugar, which not only add the right touch of sweetness but also bring their unique flavors and nutritional benefits.

The next appointment was scheduled six months later, and we analyzed the status of my health after following the treatment established previously. Subsequently, we met once a year to assess the effect of the personalized treatment. Each time, I was doing the blood, stool urine and other tests as deemed necessary by the functional medicine doctor.

Following the personalized plan, in less than 6 months, my energy improved, some of my blood tests were now within the optimum regions of the reference range and I felt alive again. From not being able to climb down the stairs from the bedroom to the living room without the need to stop for at least 30 minutes to catch my breath, I was now able to play tennis for 1-2 hours without even feeling tired. My DHEA was now optimum, my homocysteine, vitamins and minerals were showing optimum values. The gut, though, still needed some work and we started with a 21-detox program that helped me bring the liver enzymes within the desired levels. The gut is still a work in progress, and this is very important for overall physical health.

The diet did help a lot in relieving the symptoms. I pay a lot of attention to what my body tells me, and I adapt my diet accordingly. I do not use deep fried cooking methods, I prefer baked, boiled, or grilled and sometimes sauteed.

The blood tests also showed a slight descent of the thyroid markers, but they were still not within the normal values. This might be an indication that the damage to the thyroid by the autoimmune system did not progress. Same for the AIG (autoimmune gastritis markers). I don't know if they will ever go back to the levels of a healthy person, but my overall health got better, all my symptoms subsided, and all the other tests showed a big improvement which makes me believe that the progression of the disease is for now halted. As long as I keep to my diet and the new lifestyle, I am confident I can live a relatively healthy and normal life.

PART III

OUR DAY-TO-DAY POTENTIAL AUTOIMMUNE TRIGGERS

3.1 OUR LIFESTYLE

Our lives are shaped by the accumulation of days, weeks, months, and years that precede us. We are constructed from our past experiences, our spoken words, and our actions. All these elements influence our behaviors, guide our decisions, and shape the words we speak and the thoughts we think.

Our lifestyle plays a critical role in our health. What we eat, the air we breathe, the water we drink, our eating habits, the stress we endure either self-inflicted or coerced upon ourselves by the work or family problems, the pollutants we have in our homes or the chemicals we use on our skins, all impact negatively or positively how our body reacts.

In the next pages I will go over the most important aspects of our lifestyle that are negatively impacting our health:

3.1.1 OUR FOOD

Think of your diet as a financial account where every healthy food choice is a valuable investment towards your well-being.

In today's society, the abundance and accessibility of food, combined with our fast-paced lifestyle, make it tempting to opt for ready-made meals that are quick to heat and eat. However, this convenience often comes with a hidden cost to our health. Many processed foods are laden with artificial preservatives, which, in excessive amounts, can be detrimental to our well-being. Additionally, these foods often contain high levels of sodium and added sugars. Regular consumption of salt, sugar, and artificial additives, along with excessive alcohol intake and reliance on certain medications, can lay the groundwork for various health issues [84]. These dietary choices can contribute to the development of chronic diseases and overall poor health outcomes, making it imperative to be mindful of what we consume.

Sugar consumption - Recent research [85] has shed light on the profound impact of sugar on human health, drawing parallels to the way opioids affect the brain. These studies suggest that sugar can stimulate the same reward centers in the brain, leading to behavior akin to dependency. This addictive property of sugar is concerning, considering it is a common ingredient in many foods we consume daily, from bread and sauces to dairy products and even cold cuts.

The habitual consumption of sugar-rich foods and beverages can foster cravings and impulsive eating habits, a phenomenon often seen in addictive behaviors. Moreover, a diet high in sugary products, especially over extended periods, is associated with elevated levels of inflammation in the body [86]. This state of chronic inflammation is a known risk factor for a range of health issues, including the potential development of autoimmune diseases.

Understanding the impact of sugar on our health and behavior is crucial, especially in a society where sugar is ubiquitous in our food supply. Reducing sugar intake and being mindful of its presence in various food products can be an important step towards better health and reducing the risk of inflammation-related conditions.

Artificial sweeteners - Artificial sweeteners are a topic of considerable debate, especially concerning their role in weight-loss diets. While they offer a low- or zero-calorie alternative to sugar, the question remains: Are they genuinely beneficial for health? As synthetic substitutes, these sweeteners differ significantly from natural sugars, leading to concerns about their potential impact on health.

Intriguingly, research, including animal studies, has raised questions about the addictive nature of these substances. A notable example is a study highlighted in Harvard Health Publishing on January 29, 2020, where rats, previously exposed to cocaine, predominantly chose oral saccharin, an artificial sweetener, over cocaine [87]. This suggests that artificial sweeteners could potentially have an addictive quality, at least in animal models.

While artificial sweeteners are often promoted as a healthier alternative to sugar, especially for those looking to reduce calorie intake, their long-term effects on health and behavior are still being studied and understood so caution is advisable when consuming them.

Table salt - Sodium chloride, commonly known as table salt, plays a crucial role in our body's physiological functions, including the regulation of blood fluids and the maintenance of blood pressure [88]. While salt is vital for the health of the heart, liver, and kidneys, consuming it in excess can be detrimental. Excessive salt intake is associated with negative impacts on kidney health, elevated blood pressure, and an increased risk of cardiovascular diseases and stroke.

The World Health Organization (WHO) recommends limiting sodium intake to no more than 1500 mg (1.5 g) per day, roughly equivalent to half a teaspoon of table salt. This guideline is particularly important for people with diabetes, kidney stones, or cardiovascular conditions, who should be especially mindful of their sodium consumption.

A significant challenge in managing sodium intake comes from processed and canned foods, which often contain high levels of added sodium. Being aware of and tracking daily sodium consumption is crucial for maintaining health.

Furthermore, studies have indicated that high sodium intake can have addictive properties, potentially leading to increased cravings and overeating [89]. This underscores the importance of a balanced diet with careful monitoring of sodium intake, not only for physical health but also for preventing addictive eating patterns.

Food additives - According to the World Health Organization (WHO), food additives are defined as substances added to food to maintain or improve its safety, freshness, taste, texture, or appearance. These additives are broadly grouped into categories, including flavoring agents, enzyme preparations, and a variety of other additives, although there are more categories like colorants and preservatives recognized by food regulatory agencies.

Flavoring agents are a significant category, used extensively to enhance the taste of processed foods such as milk, yogurt, soft drinks, cereals, and cakes. One challenge with these agents is the lack of detailed labeling requirements. Food manufacturers are typically only required to list 'flavors' on ingredient labels without specifying the sources or composition of these flavors. This generalized labeling makes it difficult for consumers and researchers alike to evaluate the exact impact of these flavoring agents on human health.

The broad use of flavoring agents in processed foods, combined with limited transparency in labeling, raises questions about the potential health effects of these additives.

Enzyme preparations are widely used as processing aids in the food manufacturing industry, playing a crucial role in the production of baked goods, beverages, and dairy products. Enzymes, which are proteins, serve the essential function of speeding up chemical reactions, not just in food processing but also within the human body. They are vital for various bodily processes, including digestion, liver function, and muscle development.

However, when it comes to the enzymes used in food preparation, there is a relative lack of detailed information regarding their specific effects on human health. While enzymes are naturally occurring and often derived from plant or animal sources, their safety and impact in the context of food processing warrant closer examination.

In the United States, the regulation of enzymes in food manufacturing does exist under the oversight of the Food and Drug Administration (FDA). However, the regulatory framework may not be as comprehensive or stringent as it is for other food additives. This situation leads to a gap in our understanding of the long-term health implications of these enzymes when used in food processing.

Given their widespread use and the importance of enzymes in both food technology and human physiology, further research and more detailed regulatory guidelines are needed to ensure their safety and efficacy in food production. The assumption that enzymes are inherently safe due to their natural origin requires a more nuanced approach, considering the complexity of food chemistry and human health.

Artificial preservatives are ubiquitous in ready-to-eat foods, serving to extend shelf life and delay spoilage. For those looking to avoid these additives, opting for organic raw foods, which are typically free from artificial preservatives, is a viable choice.

There is a growing awareness among consumers about the potential adverse health effects of artificial preservatives. However, despite the increased scrutiny of ingredient labels, there remains a lack of widespread understanding regarding their impact on health. This is compounded by labeling practices where some harmful ingredients may be ambiguously listed under the term 'flavor.'

In particular, substances like nitrates and nitrites, often found in processed meats, have raised health concerns. In the body, they can transform into compounds with carcinogenic properties and have been linked to diseases like Alzheimer's, Parkinson's, and Type 2 diabetes. Additionally, sulfites, used in a variety of processed foods, are known to trigger severe allergic reactions in some individuals.

These concerns are highlighted in research, such as a paper published in the International Journal of Pharmaceutical Sciences and Research, which points to the need for greater awareness and caution in our food choices. When purchasing food, it is advisable to be vigilant of ingredients like nitrates/nitrites and sulfites, and to consider the broader implications of artificial preservatives on our health.

Other food additives with potential harmful effect on human's health are:

- Partially hydrogenated vegetable oil, found in cakes, cookies, soups, fast food. It contributes to heart disease.
- Yellow #5 and #6, Blue #1 & Blue #2, Red #3 and Red #40, found in cereals, chips, cookies, puddings, candy, chocolate cakes, beverages, icing. It is linked to concentration disorders in children, like ADD, potential kidneys and intestinal tumors, to cancers and thyroid tumors in rat studies.
- BHA (Butylated hydroxytoluene) and BHT (Butylated hydroxyanisole) found in beer, crackers, butter, cereals. It causes cancer in the forestomach of rats.
- Sodium phosphate, found in sausages and processed meats. It can increase the risk for heart disease.
- Corn syrup found in almost every food item from soups, meat to deserts.
- Monosodium glutamate, found in foods with meat flavoring. It causes brain-cell damage in mice.

3.1.2 CHRONIC STRESS

"If you ask what is the single most important key to longevity, I would have to say it is avoiding worry, stress and tension. And if you didn't ask me, I'd still have to say it."

George Burns, "How to Live to Be 100 - Or More.", Actor.

Our modern lifestyle, marked by a constant balancing act between personal and professional responsibilities, leads to chronic stress and anxiety, making us more susceptible to illnesses and to overeating [90]. Without effective stress management, reliance on medication with potential side effects becomes a reality.

Recent research, including a 2017 EXCLI Journal article [30], highlights how prolonged stress adversely affects various body functions, from the brain to the immune system, leading to an array of disorders. The medical community is recognizing the need for comprehensive treatment approaches, combining medication with lifestyle changes, to combat the detrimental health impacts of chronic stress.

In previous chapters I wrote more about stress and stress management.

3.1.3 OUR DIET

"Food is information. All food is not created equal. All calories are not created equal. One hundred calories of an apple, one hundred calories of pretzels behave completely differently in your body. So, unhealthy food – poor cell function, healthy food – the cells work well."

Susan Blum, MD, MPH, Functional Medicine Doctor, and Founder of Blum Center for Health

I can count on my fingers the people I met in my whole life who had good eating habits, and I have lived in 4 countries until now and met a lot of people. One of those is my husband. He does not eat more than what he needs, he does not eat in between the main meals: no snacks, no sweets, no junk food, no sweet drinks. Occasionally, he drinks one glass of wine or a beer, and that is it.

How wonderful it would be if good habits could be transmitted like a virus to or from the person next to you!

Overeating places significant stress on the stomach by causing it to expand, a response that triggers the release of more hydrochloric acid in preparation for digesting the larger quantity of food. This expansion, coupled with the additional acid, means the food remains in the stomach for an extended period, increasing the risk of irritating the stomach lining and potentially leading to gastritis.

To avoid overeating, a practical approach is to portion out the exact amount of food that constitutes a healthy meal. Once your plate is empty, resist the temptation to refill it or snack further. If you struggle with cravings, especially for sweets or other foods, try distracting yourself with activities like walking or engaging in something that diverts your attention away from food. This approach not only helps in regulating the amount of food consumed but also in managing the body's digestive response, thereby contributing to better gastrointestinal health.

Snacking, often touted as a way to boost metabolism, has become a common dietary habit. Despite recommendations by some dietitians to eat three meals a day with snacks in between, implying almost constant eating, there's limited scientific evidence to support the claim that this practice enhances metabolic rates. In fact, a meal typically takes 2 to 4 hours to move from the stomach to the small intestine [91], and frequent snacking can lead to continuously elevated glucose levels throughout the day. For those without specific medical conditions that require more frequent eating, limiting food intake to three main meals can allow the stomach to fully empty, potentially benefiting digestion.

Moreover, there's growing interest in the benefits of intermittent fasting, a practice rooted in ancient traditions across various cultures and religions. Fasting, as part of intermittent dietary patterns, has been observed to offer numerous health benefits [92].

Drinking too much alcohol - Excessive alcohol consumption poses significant risks to our health, impacting various critical systems within the body. Not only does it lead to dehydration due to its diuretic properties, but it also causes systemic damage over time. Drinking heavily in a single session or consistently over an extended period can adversely affect the heart, potentially leading to conditions like cardiomyopathy or arrhythmias. The liver, which processes alcohol, can be severely damaged, leading to cirrhosis or fatty liver disease. The pancreas is also at risk, as excessive alcohol can trigger pancreatitis, a painful and potentially dangerous condition. Additionally, regular high alcohol consumption compromises the immune system, making the body more susceptible to infections and illnesses.

The diuretic effect of alcohol further exacerbates these issues by depleting the body's water content, leading to dehydration.

Not drinking enough water - can lead to various health issues, including dehydration, fatigue, headaches, constipation, inadequate toxin elimination through urine, and dry skin. While the common belief suggests that we should drink six to eight 8-ounce glasses of water daily, the reality is that hydration needs vary from person to person. There is no universal formula that fits everyone.

A practical guideline for ensuring adequate hydration is to aim to urinate approximately every two hours. This rule of thumb considers that we also obtain fluids from other sources in our diet, such as salads, fruits, and soups, not just from drinking water. Therefore, it's important to listen to your body's signals and adjust your water intake accordingly to maintain proper hydration. Keeping track of the frequency of urination can be a helpful indicator of whether you are drinking enough fluids.

Eating your stress is a harmful habit. Turning to comfort food in times of stress, whether due to work pressures, personal relationship issues, or the loss of a loved one, is a common coping behavior. This response has been extensively studied and explained by scientists [90]. When faced with stress, our body instinctively triggers the 'fight or flight' response. This involves a shift in bodily functions: activities like digestion, reproduction, and tissue repair are slowed down, while heart rate, blood pressure, and breathing are accelerated. The body is effectively preparing for immediate physical action in response to perceived danger.

In situations of short-term stress, these automatic changes are beneficial, helping us to quickly react and escape from immediate threats. However, when stress becomes chronic, the scenario changes. The adrenal glands continue to release cortisol, a stress hormone, which remains elevated. This increase in cortisol boosts both appetite and the motivation to eat, even when we're not actually hungry. As a result, we often find ourselves eating in response to stress rather than hunger, placing additional strain on our digestive system and overall bodily health. This pattern of 'eating your stress' can lead to a cycle of overeating and may contribute to various health issues over time.

3.1.4 EXERCISE (OR BETTER SAID THE LACK OF EXERCISE)

> *"The doctor of the future will give no medicine but will involve the patient in the proper use of food, fresh air, and exercise."*
>
> *Thomas Edison, Innovator, and businessman*

Unfortunately, Thomas Edison's vision has not yet come true.

Recommending physical activity to sustain good health has roots in antiquity. More than 2400 years ago, a physician from India, Susruta, the father of surgery, was the first to prescribe "moderate daily exercise" [93] to his patients and later on Hippocrates, the father of modern medicine, wrote "eating alone will not keep a man well; he must also take exercise." [94].

It is intuitive to associate sedentarism with a long list of diseases like obesity, cardiovascular problems, high blood pressure, high cholesterol, cancer, depression, anxiety. It is less intuitive to make a connection between sedentarism and autoimmune diseases. Recent studies have shown that regular exercise should be part of the strategy to manage autoimmune diseases [95] since it helps reduce the inflammation in our bodies, it improves circulation of the oxygen to all the cells, and it improves brain function.

In modern times sedentarism took a different meaning than living in one place for a long time and became a plague affecting our health. Sedentarism is defined as the activities that are performed sitting or lying down, like reading, watching TV, working in front of a computer, etc. with little or no physical movement. It is estimated that "Approximately 31% of the global population aged ≥15 years engages in insufficient physical activity, and it is known to contribute to the death of approximately 3.2 million people every year" [96].

So how much moderate intensity exercise do we must do to keep a healthy life? Different countries have different recommendations: the Australian Government Department of Health recommends 150-300 minutes per week for adults; in South Korea the recommendation is to limit the sedentary activities to 2 hours per day and engage the rest of the time in low level physical activity; in USA, the American College of Sports Medicine recommends 30 minutes of exercise, five days a week therefore, a 150 minutes per week.

If we want to be healthy or to keep at bay a chronic, autoimmune disease we must be mindful and stop a sedentary activity every 2 hours, take a few steps to help the blood circulation and the oxygenation of our cells and brain. We also must engage in a crisp walking or other medium impact exercise permitted by our individual situation at least 30 minutes per day.

3.1.5 SLEEP

Sleep is good medicine, when our physical body heals, and our mind gets organized.

I know! You will tell me "We sleep one third of our lives, so if we are lucky and live to be 90 years old, we slept 30 years. So, why not cut down on sleeping hours?".

Sleep deprivation significantly undermines our health, as sleep is the time when our body actively engages in repairing cells and tissues. Everyone's sleep needs are unique, but generally, adults require about seven to eight hours of sleep each night for optimal functioning during the day. It's not just the duration of sleep that matters, but also its quality.

While we sleep, we alternate between two critical phases: Rapid Eye Movement (REM) and non-Rapid Eye Movement (non-REM) sleep, cycling through these stages several times each night. During non-REM sleep, particularly in its deeper stages, the body enters a state of relaxation. Heart rate, body temperature, and breathing slow down, muscles relax, and the body focuses on physical healing and recovery. This phase is crucial for physical rejuvenation, allowing us to recover from the day's stress and strains. Meanwhile, REM sleep, known for its characteristic eye movements, plays a vital role in brain functions like memory consolidation and processing emotions.

Understanding and prioritizing both the quantity and quality of our sleep is essential for maintaining overall health and well-being, as it's a time when our body and mind undergo essential restorative processes.

Deficient sleep has significant adverse effects on health, notably increasing vulnerability to infections and potentially leading to inflammatory and autoimmune diseases [97]. The immune system, complex in its functioning, relies on adequate sleep for optimal performance. When deprived of sufficient sleep, our body produces fewer antibodies, diminishing its ability to fend off viruses, bacteria, and other pathogens. This weakened immune response not only makes us more susceptible to infections but also increases inflammation, which can contribute to cardiovascular and metabolic diseases. Additionally, the reduced activity of immune cells capable of targeting tumor cells or virus-infected cells heightens the risk of viral infections and potentially, cancer.

Another consequence of sleep deprivation is an increase in appetite, which can lead to obesity. This issue is often compounded by the types of food consumed during extended waking hours, which can exacerbate inflammation. This creates a vicious cycle of metabolic changes driven by both the physiological effects of sleep loss and lifestyle factors, such as prolonged waking hours leading to increased food intake and heightened stress levels.

3.2 PRESCRIPTION MEDICATIONS

"The person who takes medicine must recover twice, once from the disease and once from the medicine."

William Osler, Physician, one of the four founding professors of Johns Hopkins Hospital, "The Father of Modern Medicine".

In previous chapters I wrote about the danger of side effects of prescription medication. Since this is an important subject given the ease with which the medication is prescribed for hiding the symptoms I will continue spending a little bit of time here too.

In reflecting on the role of prescription medication in modern healthcare, I am reminded of the historical context of pain management. Before the advent of drugs like Tylenol and Advil, people had to rely on natural remedies and endure more pain. There's no denying the remarkable achievements of modern medicine: eradicating diseases like polio, tuberculosis, and Ebola; significantly increasing life expectancy; reducing infant and maternal mortality; and making day-to-day life more bearable for many suffering from various ailments. These advances are particularly evident in emergency care and in treating acute conditions.

However, this progress should not overshadow certain realities. Today, despite longer lifespans and better management of pain, it doesn't necessarily equate to overall better health compared to earlier times. We live longer, but this extended life isn't always accompanied by improved health, partly due to the overuse or mismanagement of prescription medications. In some cases, the side effects of these medications can lead to additional health complications, creating a paradox where treatment might contribute to further health decline.

Due to our lifestyle and the food that we eat, I see more and more of my friends and acquaintances turning towards medication to deal with a heartburn or with a general pain. Having the medication readily available over the counter does not make things better for the normal person who trusts the system and believes that if the medication is so available it is because it is helpful and cannot do any harm. Even worse is when a physician is prescribing medication for ailments that can be cured (yes, you heard me right: CURED) by changing our lifestyles: diets, sleep patterns, stress control, clean environment, exercise.

Have you ever wondered how the medical field transitioned from primarily prescribing herbs and diet-based treatments in the early 1900s to the pharmaceutical-centric approach we see today? A key figure in this transition was John D. Rockefeller (1839 – 1937), America's first billionaire and a major player in the oil industry who controlled 90% of the oil refineries in the U.S. When the ability of creating chemicals from oil was invented, he saw a golden mine in developing pharmaceutical drugs out of oil. He monopolized the oil and pharmaceutical industries.

But he also needed to redefine the medicine to sell the newly invented drugs. So, he started to lobby to modernize the medical institutions. Rockefeller's investments in medical colleges and hospitals played a role in shaping modern medical education and practices. He contributed significantly to funding medical research and institutions, which influenced the direction of medical science and training. Legal actions against medical practitioners who were promoting homeopathy and natural remedies during this period were related to this type of practice considered fraudulent or harmful under the emerging medical standards. He also founded the American Cancer Society which is "healing" people with chemotherapy and more drugs. Nowadays, doctors are practicing medicine as it was modified to suit the interests of Rockefeller and the pharmaceutical companies, in which a pill is the answer to any diagnosis.

We need to recognize that prescription drugs, many of which are synthetic, all come with potential side effects. It's important to understand that these side effects can sometimes be quite significant, potentially presenting more challenges than the original condition they're meant to treat. It's a delicate balance that healthcare providers and patients must navigate, taking into account the seriousness of the condition being treated and the individual patient's health profile. Informed decision-making and close monitoring are key to ensuring that the therapeutic benefits of medication outweigh the potential adverse effects.

Despite accumulating evidence and longstanding knowledge that diet and lifestyle are crucial in preventing and managing diseases like type 2 diabetes, heart conditions, and certain cancers [98], there is a notable gap in medical education concerning nutrition. As it stands, only about "one-fifth of American medical schools require their students to take a nutrition course" [99]. This shortfall in nutrition education is concerning, given the critical role that diet plays in health and disease management. While there's a growing recognition of this issue and some medical schools are beginning to address it, the integration of comprehensive nutrition training into medical curriculum remains a significant challenge that needs more attention in the healthcare education system.

"Today, most medical schools in the United States teach less than 25 hours of nutrition over four years. The fact that less than 20 percent of medical schools have a single required course in nutrition, it's a scandal. It's outrageous. It's obscene," says David Eisenberg, adjunct associate professor of nutrition at Harvard T.H. Chan School of Public Health [99]

It's disheartening to reflect on my experiences with the healthcare system regarding prescription medication, particularly PPIs, statins (I am continuously pushed to take them for my elevated "bad" cholesterol despite latest studies showing the opposite) and antidepressants (since I am stubborn and challenge the doctors in in trying to understand the reason for my symptoms). When I inquired about its side effects back in 2009, my gastroenterologist assured me of its safety, even comparing it favorably to birth control pills. This sentiment was echoed by other GI specialists I consulted with until 2015. However, by the end of 2015, concerns about PPI's long-term safety began to surface, including links to stomach cancer, kidney failure, and other serious health issues, leading to a class-action lawsuit. When I challenged my GI doctor about the possibility of discontinuing the PPIs, I was met with a dismissive response, without further explanation and prescribed antidepressants.

It is important to understand that there is no chemical pill without side effects. The doctors should prescribe first lifestyle changes (diet, stress reductions activities, exercise) as much as possible and leave the use of pills only when there is no other option.

Due to Rockefeller, today's healthcare is not focused on a cure but on the symptoms which bring more customers and ensures keeping the current ones by creating drug addictions or other illnesses that require new drugs.

I will leave the subject of prescription medication with the words of Peter C Gotzsche, a Danish physician, medical researcher, and leader of the Nordic Cochrane Centre at Rigshospitalet in Copenhagen, Denmark [23]:

"Our prescription drugs are the third leading cause of death after heart disease and cancer (1). Based on the best research I could find, I have estimated that psychiatric drugs alone are also the third major killer (2), mainly because antidepressants kill many elderly people through falls (3). This tells us that the system we have for researching, approving, marketing, and using drugs is totally broken (1,2)."

3.3 OUR ENVIRONMENT

"It is our collective and individual responsibility to preserve and tend to the world in which we all live."

Dalai Lama, Spiritual Leader

The environment in which we live is a critical determinant of our health. In recent times, there's been an increasing focus on the challenges posed by climate change and the imperative to control air pollution. These environmental issues are not just about preserving the planet but are directly linked to our health and survival as human beings.

3.3.1 AIR QUALITY

In urban environments, the quality of air, often compromised by various pollutants, chemicals, and allergens, is a primary factor in triggering asthma and other serious breathing symptoms for many individuals.

Air pollution is a serious concern, and is associated with different diseases like lung cancers, cardiovascular diseases, respiratory problems like asthma, chronic bronchitis, and others. The World Health Organization (WHO) estimated in 2021 that approximately 4.2 million people die annually due to outside air pollution and 3.8 million people die annually due to indoor air pollution [101]. In the USA, the number of deaths caused by air quality was estimated at 60,200 in 2019 [102]. The biggest offenders that have a negative effect on our health are the very small particles that are airborne, like sulfates, nitrates, mineral dust, black carbon, and others, called under the generic name Particulate Matter (PM) that cannot be seen with the naked eye. These particles get into our lungs and into our bloodstream and therefore into all our body. If it is difficult for each of us to control the outside air quality, it is easier to control the air quality inside our homes. Since most of us spend more time indoors, it makes sense to affirm that the risks of being exposed to polluted air is greater indoors than outdoors.

Indoor air quality is significantly influenced by a variety of common elements, each carrying potential health risks. Among these are smoke from tobacco and wood-burning stoves, which can release a range of harmful particles and gasses into the air. These particles can aggravate respiratory conditions like asthma and bronchitis and long-term exposure can increase the risk of more serious lung diseases.

Carbon monoxide, a colorless and odorless gas, is another harmful byproduct often found indoors, typically emitted from fireplaces, furnaces, boilers, and gas or wood stoves. Exposure to high levels of carbon monoxide can be life-threatening, causing symptoms like headaches, dizziness, and, in extreme cases, can lead to carbon monoxide poisoning.

Building materials, particularly in older constructions, can be sources of indoor pollution. Insulation containing asbestos, for instance, poses significant health risks. Asbestos fibers, when disturbed and inhaled, can lead to lung diseases, including asbestosis and mesothelioma. Radon, a naturally occurring radioactive gas that can seep into buildings from the ground, is another critical concern. It's a leading cause of lung cancer among non-smokers.

Molds, which thrive in damp environments, can adversely affect indoor air quality. Exposure to mold spores can trigger allergic reactions, respiratory issues, and in severe cases, lead to more serious health problems, especially in individuals with compromised immune systems.

Furthermore, products like air fresheners, often used to improve the scent of indoor spaces, can emit a variety of chemicals that might irritate the lungs and exacerbate respiratory issues, especially when used excessively.

Alongside the previously mentioned indoor air pollutants, new furniture treatments contribute significantly to indoor air quality concerns. Furniture and upholstery are often treated with various chemicals for different purposes — be it for fire resistance, stain-proofing, or to prevent the growth of microbes. These treatments can release volatile organic compounds (VOCs) into the air, which are known to have adverse health effects.

VOCs are a group of chemicals that easily evaporate at room temperature and can be emitted by a wide range of products used in homes and offices, including new furniture. Exposure to VOCs can lead to a variety of short-term health effects such as headaches, dizziness, eye, nose, and throat irritation, as well as more severe long-term effects like liver, kidney, or central nervous system damage. Some VOCs are also suspected or known to cause cancer in humans.

The 'off-gassing' of these chemicals is most potent when the furniture is new and can diminish over time. However, the initial period after bringing new furniture into a home or office can be particularly concerning in terms of air quality. It's vital to ensure adequate ventilation during this time to disperse these compounds more effectively. Additionally, seeking out furniture that is certified to have low or no VOC emissions can also be a prudent step in reducing overall exposure to these harmful chemicals.

The impact of these pollutants can range from immediate effects like headaches and respiratory discomfort to long-term health consequences, including chronic respiratory diseases and cancer. The effects might be more pronounced after prolonged or repeated exposure, highlighting the importance of proactive measures. These include improving ventilation, using air purifiers, maintaining heating and cooking appliances, controlling humidity to prevent mold growth, and using building and cleaning materials that are safer and less toxic.

The U.S. Environmental Protection Agency (EPA) and the U.S. Consumer Product Safety Commission (CSPC) have information regarding the steps we can take to reduce the pollution in our homes.

3.3.2 WATER QUALITY

Water quality is not just a matter of health – it's a matter of survival.

The consumption of contaminated water is a significant global health concern, linked to the transmission of diseases such as diarrhea, dysentery, hepatitis A, cholera, and polio.

Daily hydration plays a critical role in maintaining our bodily functions. While the recommended daily water intake can vary based on individual needs, lifestyle, and climate, a general guideline is to consume between 4 and 8 cups of water per day. This helps in multiple ways: it aids in preventing kidney stones, which can occur due to concentrated urine; it alleviates constipation by aiding bowel movements; it helps maintain clear cognition, as even mild dehydration can impair mental function; and it regulates body temperature, preventing overheating.

Beyond personal consumption, water is integral in various aspects of daily life, including cooking and hygiene. Hence, the cleanliness of water used in cooking and cleaning is equally important.

To ensure the water we use is clean and not life-threatening, it's essential to implement and maintain effective water treatment and sanitation systems. At the individual level, using home water filters, boiling water, or using bottled water (in areas where tap water safety is questionable) can be practical steps.

A lot of people are under the impression that bottled water is better than tap water. If you are one of them, I will have to ask you to take a few minutes and think about the plastic in which the bottled water is coming from and the effect of different chemicals released in the water by the plastic bottle exposed to high heat or cold while transportation and refrigeration. A study made in 2018 on 259 individual bottles from 11 different brands, from 19 locations in nine different countries found a staggering 93% contamination rate with microplastics. A little more than half (54%) of these microplastics particles were confirmed to be polypropylene which is used for the manufacturing of the bottle caps and another 4% showing the presence of industrial lubricants. This discovery is alarming, particularly as these particles are primarily derived from the bottles themselves and the bottling process. Intriguingly, the level of microplastic contamination in bottled water was found to be almost double that of tap water from the same regions, raising significant health concerns [103].

While research on the impact of microplastics on human health is ongoing, animal studies suggest potential risks. These small particles have been found to accumulate in vital organs, potentially leading to toxicity and adverse health effects [104]. This ongoing research is critical in understanding the long-term implications of consuming microplastics through bottled water.

Turning to tap water, its safety generally depends on the local water supply and infrastructure. In many areas of the USA, Canada, and Europe, public water systems provide safe drinking water. However, this water is not without its challenges. Tap water is commonly treated with chlorine and other chemicals to eliminate pathogens, but these substances can affect water taste and quality. Furthermore, aging infrastructure can lead to additional contaminants entering the water supply. Old pipes, for example, might leach lead or other harmful metals into the water, posing serious health risks. In regions where water quality may be compromised, using home water filtration systems can be a practical solution. These filters can remove a range of contaminants, including chlorine byproducts, heavy metals, and even microplastics, improving the safety and taste of the water.

The environmental impact of bottled water also extends beyond the issue of microplastics. The production and disposal of plastic bottles contribute significantly to environmental pollution and resource depletion. Conversely, tap water has a lower environmental footprint, although infrastructure and maintenance issues can present challenges.

When considering the choice between bottled and tap water, it's essential to weigh the health risks, environmental impacts, and local water quality. Understanding these factors can help individuals make informed decisions about their water consumption, whether it's opting for filtered tap water or selecting bottled water brands with rigorous quality control measures.

If you want to know how good the water in your area is, you can find out by surfing the Environmental Working Group (ewg) website www.ewg.org/tapwater/.

3.3.3 MOLDS

"Air, water and places."

Hippocrates, Ancient Greek physician

With the above Hippocrates reminds us that, while our understanding of specific health risks has evolved, the fundamental principle of environmental influence on health remains unchanged.

Molds are a diverse group of fungi that can be found in various environments, both indoors and outdoors. They grow on organic materials such as wood, drywall, plants, and food. One of the key characteristics of mold is its ability to release spores, which are tiny, lightweight, and easily become airborne. These airborne spores can be inhaled by individuals, leading to various health problems.

Health Impacts of Mold Exposure:

- **Allergic Reactions:** Common symptoms include a runny nose, sneezing, watery eyes, and skin irritation. These reactions are particularly prevalent in individuals with mold allergies.
- **Respiratory Issues:** Mold exposure can exacerbate asthma and other respiratory conditions, causing symptoms like coughing, wheezing, and difficulty breathing.
- **Severe Health Effects:** Prolonged exposure to high levels of mold can lead to more serious health issues, including headaches, chronic fatigue, and respiratory infections. In some cases, it can cause toxic effects due to mycotoxins produced by certain types of molds.

Growth Conditions and Prevention:

- **Moisture Control:** Since mold requires moisture to grow, controlling humidity levels is crucial. This can be achieved through proper ventilation, use of dehumidifiers, and

addressing any water leaks or condensation issues promptly.
- **Temperature Regulation:** While it's challenging to maintain temperatures outside the mold-friendly range in typical home environments, regulating indoor temperature can help reduce the risk of mold growth.
- **Regular Cleaning:** Regularly cleaning areas prone to moisture, such as bathrooms and kitchens, can prevent mold buildup. It's also important to keep fabrics and carpets dry and well-maintained.

Common Locations in Homes:

- **High Humidity Areas:** Bathrooms, basements, and kitchens are common mold growth areas due to their typically higher humidity levels.
- **HVAC Systems:** Molds can thrive in air conditioning and heating systems, particularly in ducts where dust and moisture can accumulate.
- **Hidden Spots:** Molds can grow in less visible places like behind wallpaper, under carpets, inside wall cavities, or around plumbing pipes, making them harder to detect and address.

Apart from health concerns, mold can cause significant damage to the structure of buildings. Prolonged exposure to mold can weaken wooden structures, degrade drywall, and damage other building materials.

Recognizing the signs of mold in your home is crucial for timely intervention. Key indicators include:

- **Distinct Odor:** A damp, musty smell is often the first sign of mold. This odor is caused by chemicals emitted by the mold as it grows and spreads.
- **Visual Clues:** Look for spots or stains on carpets, walls, or ceilings, which might indicate moisture problems and mold growth. In areas like bathrooms, kitchens, and laundry rooms, dark spots in tile grout or around fixtures such as tubs and showers can also signal mold.
- **Health Symptoms:** Pay attention to changes in health

among household members. Mycotoxins, harmful substances produced by certain molds, can cause a range of symptoms from sneezing and coughing to fatigue and more serious allergic reactions. These symptoms can be especially pronounced in individuals with mold sensitivities or respiratory conditions.

The severity of symptoms often correlates with the concentration of mold and the duration of exposure. If you or someone in your household experiences these symptoms, and you suspect mold might be the cause, it's advisable to consult a mold specialist for a thorough evaluation of your home. Professional assessment is essential, as mold can sometimes grow in hidden areas, making it difficult to detect and remove without expert help.

3.4 OUR EVERYDAY CHEMICALS EXPOSURE

Everywhere we look, we are surrounded in our everyday lives by chemical products. When it comes to using cleaning, skin care products or fragrances the best rule is if it's not coming from a natural source, don't use it.

3.4.1 HOUSEHOLD CLEANING PRODUCTS

By conducting a chemical cleanse of your living space, you and your children can avoid unknowingly participating in a large-scale, real-world experiment with dangerous outcomes for your health.

In our efforts to maintain clean and germ-free homes, we often rely on household chemicals, unaware that this practice might be detrimental to our health rather than beneficial. Research has established a clear connection between the use of common cleaning agents, such as bleach, glass cleaners, air fresheners, and detergents, and respiratory issues. Notably, there has been an observed increase in asthma cases, particularly among women who engage in regular cleaning activities. However, the impact of these chemicals extends beyond the lungs, affecting various other organs and systems including the thyroid, immune system, liver, hormonal system, and skin, potentially leading to autoimmune disorders.

The health risks associated with the chemical exposure to cleaning products are:

- **Toxic Ingredients:** Many cleaning products contain harmful chemicals like ammonia, bleach, and formaldehyde.

Prolonged exposure to these chemicals can lead to respiratory issues, skin irritation, and allergic reactions. Certain chemicals found in cleaning agents have been linked to more serious health issues, including cancer and hormone disruption.

- **Asthma and Respiratory Problems:** Sprays, aerosols, and other volatile products can contribute to indoor air pollution. They release harmful particles and chemicals into the air, which can trigger asthma attacks and exacerbate respiratory conditions. People with pre-existing respiratory issues are particularly at risk.

- **Skin and Eye Irritation:** Direct contact with cleaning products can cause skin and eye irritation. Some ingredients in these products can be corrosive, leading to burns or rashes. Wearing gloves and eye protection is recommended when using these products.

- **Accidental Poisoning:** Accidental ingestion or improper use of household cleaners can lead to poisoning, especially in children and pets. Keeping these products out of reach and following the usage instructions is critical to prevent accidental poisoning.

Apart from health risks, many cleaning products have a detrimental effect on the environment. Chemicals washed down the drain can contaminate water sources and harm aquatic life. The production and disposal of plastic containers for these products contribute to environmental pollution and resource depletion.

The COVID-19 pandemic has further exacerbated this issue, with a marked rise in the use of hand sanitizers and disinfectants. These products are frequently applied to the skin and inhaled during use, posing additional health risks. This situation is particularly concerning given the vast number of chemicals in circulation. As noted by the Natural Resources Defense Council (NRDC), out of over 80,000 chemicals currently used in the United States, the majority have not undergone sufficient testing for their effects on human health [105].

It's crucial to recognize that one does not need to wait until experiencing chemical sensitivity or developing an autoimmune disease to become proactive. Educating oneself about the potential hazards of these cleaning products and seeking out non-toxic alternatives is a vital step towards preserving our health and wellbeing. This approach not only benefits individual health but also contributes to a safer environment, as many of these chemicals can have adverse environmental impacts as well. Therefore, it is imperative to be mindful of the cleaning products we choose and to consider their long-term effects on our health and the planet.

When using cleaning products, it is better to look for safer alternatives such as:

- **Natural and Eco-friendly Products:** Using natural cleaning products made from ingredients like vinegar, baking soda, and lemon juice can be a safer alternative. These products are less likely to cause health issues and are better for the environment.

- **Proper Ventilation:** Ensuring good ventilation when using cleaning products can reduce the risk of respiratory problems. Open windows or use fans to circulate fresh air.

- **Reading Labels Carefully:** Being informed about the ingredients and proper usage of cleaning products can help minimize health risks. Look for products with fewer chemical ingredients and clear safety instructions.

- **Safe Storage and Usage:** Store cleaning products safely and use them according to the manufacturer's instructions. Keep them away from children and pets to prevent accidental ingestion.

3.4.2 SKIN CARE PRODUCTS

"Personal care products expose children to an average of 60 chemicals every day that they can breathe in or absorb through their skin."

The Environmental Working Group (EWG)

Skincare products, an integral part of daily grooming routines for many, promise benefits like improved skin appearance and protection. However, they often contain chemicals that can pose significant health risks, including the potential to trigger autoimmune diseases.

Most of the skincare products have toxic ingredients such as:

- **Harmful Chemicals:** Skincare items, including moisturizers, sunscreens, makeup, and anti-aging creams, often contain parabens, phthalates, formaldehyde, and sulfates. These substances can disrupt hormonal balance and cause skin irritation, with some linked to serious health issues like cancer.

- **Skin Irritation and Allergies:** These products can cause allergic reactions and skin irritations, ranging from mild redness to severe dermatitis, especially in individuals with sensitive skin.

- **Sunscreen Chemicals:** Chemicals like oxybenzone and octinoxate in sunscreens, while protecting against UV radiation, can be absorbed into the skin and disrupt hormonal balance.

- **Nanoparticles:** Common in skincare for their transparent application, nanoparticles such as micronized zinc oxide and titanium oxide can penetrate the skin and enter the bloodstream, potentially causing oxidative stress and cellular damage.

As previously described, autoimmune diseases result from chronic inflammation in the body. The skin, being the largest organ, is a primary defense against hazardous substances. However, many skincare products contain nanoparticles that, when applied to the skin, can penetrate the barrier and enter the bloodstream. These particles, found in products like sun creams, lotions, facial creams, and even nail polish, can lead to inflammation, a precursor to autoimmune diseases. In the case of nail polish, the nanoparticles can even be inhaled while applying it and it can stay in the lungs and other organs even six months after the inhalation [106]. Nanoparticles that cross the skin barrier and get into the bloodstream or into the lungs by inhalation lead to inflammation which may lead in the long run to autoimmune diseases. This regular exposure to foreign substances in skincare products can lead the immune system to become overactive, attacking the body itself.

Chronic use of these products can lead to cumulative exposure to harmful chemicals, contributing to long-term health issues. Additionally, the environmental impact of these products, from the chemicals entering waterways to the pollution from packaging, is significant.

If using skincare products, consider safer alternatives and practices:

- **Natural and Organic Products**: Choosing products with natural ingredients can reduce exposure to harmful chemicals.

- **Label Awareness**: Understanding ingredient lists helps in avoiding products with known harmful chemicals.

- **Patch Testing and Professional Consultation**: Testing new products and consulting skincare professionals can minimize risks of adverse reactions.

3.4.3 DENTAL AMALGAMS

Dental amalgams, primarily mercury-based and popular for their affordability and durability, pose potential health risks due to mercury exposure, leading to a gradual shift towards alternative materials with unknown long-term effects.

Dental amalgams, a staple in dental restorative practices since the 19th century, have been the subject of ongoing health debates. Initially, gold and mercury amalgam were the materials of choice for filling dental cavities. However, due to the high cost of gold, mercury amalgam, a more affordable option, gained widespread popularity, especially for back teeth where aesthetics is less of a concern.

Mercury amalgam, a mixture of mercury and other metals, is prized for its ease of mixing, placement, and molding into tooth cavities. It hardens quickly into a durable material capable of withstanding the forces of mastication. Despite its practical benefits, concerns about the health effects of mercury exposure have persisted.

The primary concern with dental amalgams is the release of mercury vapor, especially during placement, wear and tear over time, or removal of fillings. Inhaling mercury vapor leads to its absorption into the bloodstream, potentially affecting various organs and systems.

While governmental and non-governmental studies specifically investigating the health impact of mercury amalgams have been inconclusive, general research on mercury exposure indicates links with inflammation, autoantibodies, and renal pathology [107,108]. Mercury's toxic nature raises concerns about its systemic effects on human health.

Recently, alternatives such as composite materials, glass ionomer cements, and other hybrid structures have been developed, particularly for front teeth where aesthetics are crucial. These materials do not contain mercury, but there is limited information on their long-term health impacts.

While some countries have limited or phased out the use of dental amalgams, others continue their use, citing a lack of conclusive evidence against their safety. The FDA considers them safe for most of the population, but the debate continues in the dental community.

The best way to avoid any toxic, potentially harmful material in our mouth is to keep good dental hygiene and keep away from refined sugars.

CONCLUSION

Despite the discoveries done in the last century in the field of medicine, the intricacies of our physical body still remain a puzzle for medical professionals. Presently, our economy is predominantly governed by a pursuit of substantial financial gains. Within the food industry, the use of inexpensive ingredients is prevalent to maximize profits, accompanied by the incorporation of harmful preservatives and colorants to prolong product shelf life. Additionally, the strategic inclusion of sugar and salt aims to cultivate addiction to specific tastes.

Meanwhile, the pharmaceutical industry exerts control over the protocols followed and the medications prescribed for various ailments. This dynamic often results in the provision of food that adversely impacts our health, fostering addiction. Consequently, individuals may find themselves prescribed medications to mitigate the ensuing symptoms. This cyclic pattern could potentially contribute to the emergence of further health issues, leading to the need for additional medication.

Every medication or supplement inevitably comes with potential side effects. Recognizing the essential need for a specific medication is crucial in making informed decisions about its use.

Functional medicine guides us to rediscover the significance of natural food, stress management, the impact of toxins that have infiltrated our lives over the past century, and the role of exercise. It underscores the importance of identifying the root cause and tailoring treatments based on data from diagnostic tests rather than solely addressing symptoms.

I gained firsthand insight into the profound impact of psychological stress on our physical health. I discovered that our well-being is intricately linked to our dietary choices, emphasizing the importance of considering the diet of the animals we consume therefore choosing organic and grass fed over other options. Additionally, I became aware of the potential harm posed by environmental chemicals present in water, furniture, cosmetics, shampoo, soap, and more. This journey taught me the crucial skill of tuning into and listening to my body.

I've come to recognize the importance of heeding my intuition when it signals that something isn't right. I've also learned not to fear or feel ashamed about seeking second or even third opinions if necessary. Understanding that doctors don't possess the absolute truth and that their specialization may limit their perspective on the overall impact of treatments has been an eye-opening realization.

Taking charge of my health has become a priority, realizing the need to be my own advocate. I've embraced the truth that knowledge is power, prompting me to engage in continuous study to comprehend the latest medical discoveries. It's crucial to question doctors when their approach seems solely focused on prescribing medication.

Furthermore, I've discovered that making changes to one's diet and lifestyle is indeed challenging but entirely achievable.

The human body functions as a holistic system and disrupting one component affects the equilibrium of the entire system. It's essential to recognize that true health involves maintaining a balance not only within the body but also between the mind and soul.

In my quest to understand what went wrong with my health and how I can stop the evolution of my ailment I got to discover Functional Medicine which I believe is, for now, the answer to treating chronic diseases.

In the last decade, several groundbreaking discoveries and advancements in the field of medicine and health have offered deeper insights into the complex interplay of genetic, environmental, and lifestyle factors in influencing individual health and disease processes.

These advancements have collectively contributed to the growth and development of Functional Medicine, enabling practitioners to better understand and treat the underlying causes of disease in a more holistic and individualized manner.

While Functional Medicine offers valuable insights and approaches to healthcare, its full integration into conventional medicine is hindered by differing philosophies, evidentiary standards, educational frameworks, and systemic structures.

For acute disease management, conventional medicine excels with its well-established protocols, quick interventions, and advanced emergency care techniques. In contrast, for prevention and chronic disease management, Functional Medicine is often more effective due to its holistic, personalized approach that focuses on underlying causes and long-term lifestyle and dietary modifications.

I learned that proactivity in managing your health is crucial to preventing harmful effects and various health issues. Our unique identities are shaped by a myriad of factors: our life experiences, the environment in which we were raised, our families, and our communities. Our health is also the culmination of our life choices – the food we eat, how we manage stress. Often, we opt for convenience, choosing fast food or quick-fix medications for immediate relief from issues like heartburn or bloating, without considering the long-term side effects. Developing a chronic disease is a gradual process; thus, restoring our body to a state of balance is equally gradual and requires time and effort. There's no miracle cure devoid of side effects. Adopting a healthy lifestyle – encompassing nutritious eating, proper sleep, effective stress management, and a holistic mind-body approach – is essential in managing chronic conditions. It's important to recognize that while medications might alleviate symptoms, they do not cure underlying chronic conditions such as leaky gut or autoimmune diseases. Our journey towards health is a personal one, and it's crucial to take an active role in guiding our bodies back to equilibrium and wellness.

PART IV

THE DIET

4.1 DIFFERENT FACETS OF HEALTH

Throughout the various stages of our lives, each of us stands as a distinct individual with specific needs that evolve over time.

As a Certified Integrative Nutrition Health Coach, my approach recognizes that human beings are inherently complex, consisting of multiple dimensions that collectively influence our overall health. We are not just physical entities but bio-individual beings, each with a unique constitution that requires a personalized approach to health and well-being.

Our health is a tapestry woven from various threads: physical, mental, emotional, and spiritual. Each dimension plays a crucial role in shaping our quality of life and cannot be addressed in isolation.

- **Physical Health**: It includes our dietary habits, physical activity levels, genetic predispositions, and the impact of our lifestyle choices. Nutritional choices, for instance, affect our energy levels, weight, and vulnerability to chronic diseases, while regular physical activity strengthens our bodies and enhances our mood.

- **Mental Health**: Our mental state, shaped by our thoughts, beliefs, and attitudes, significantly influences our overall well-being. A positive mindset, resilience to stress, and effective coping mechanisms are essential for mental and emotional stability.

- **Emotional Health**: This aspect involves our ability to form healthy relationships, express emotions appropriately, and manage the inevitable challenges of daily life. Emotional health is characterized by self-awareness, empathy, and the capacity to navigate complex social dynamics.

- **Spiritual Health**: Often overlooked in conventional health paradigms, spiritual well-being reflects our values, sense of purpose, and connection to a higher power or broader existence. Whether through religion, meditation, or nature, nurturing our spiritual health provides a foundation for resilience and contentment.

The principle of bio-individuality acknowledges that there is no one-size-fits-all solution to health. Each person's unique genetic makeup, environmental exposures, and life experiences dictate their specific health needs and how they respond to different diets, lifestyles, and treatments. Personalization is key; what works for one individual may not work for another. This individual variance demands that health strategies be flexible, adaptable, and tailored to the individual's changing needs over time.

Incorporating these principles into practice involves a holistic assessment of an individual's life and health, followed by the development of customized strategies that address the full spectrum of health dimensions. Through this approach, it is possible to support individuals in achieving optimal health, vitality, and fulfillment.

Now that we have a deeper insight into the interconnectedness of various health dimensions and the importance of recognizing and catering to the unique needs of each individual for optimal health we can discuss the complex subject of Diet.

4.2 WHAT IS A DIET?

Eat to live and not live to eat.

The definition of Diet is the sum of food and drink a person or a group of people consume. Many people associate the word diet with a meal regimen designed to lose weight. In reality, a diet is not merely about restriction or the pursuit of weight loss but encompasses a wide range of practices and philosophies regarding food consumption. It is a personalized and dynamic concept that can change over an individual's lifetime based on health goals, ethical beliefs, cultural practices, and personal preferences.

A diet can be understood from multiple perspectives, depending on the context in which it is discussed:

- **Nutritional Aspect:** At its most basic, a diet refers to the sum of food consumed by a person or other organism. This definition emphasizes the nutritional intake and its composition, including carbohydrates, fats, proteins, vitamins, minerals, and water, which are necessary for maintaining life and health.

- **Health and Medical Aspect:** In a health context, a diet often pertains to a specific intake of nutrition for health or weight-management reasons. Diets can be prescribed for medical conditions, such as diabetes or heart disease, where certain foods must be consumed or avoided to manage the condition effectively.

- **Weight Management:** Popularly, the term diet is associated with the use of specific food intake strategies to lose, gain, or maintain weight. This can include calorie restriction, macronutrient balancing, and the elimination or reduction of certain food groups.

- **Cultural and Lifestyle Aspect:** Diets can also reflect personal, ethical, or cultural preferences. Examples include vegetarian, vegan, ketogenic, paleo, and Mediterranean diets, among others. These dietary patterns are often adopted as part of an individual's lifestyle and can be influenced by ethical beliefs, health concerns, or cultural practices.

- **Ecological Aspect:** Some diets are chosen based on environmental sustainability and ethical considerations regarding animal welfare and ecological impact. These might prioritize locally sourced, organic, or plant-based foods to minimize the individual's carbon footprint and environmental impact.

It is believed that there are over 100 diets, but the exact real number is difficult to quantify due to the continuous emergence of new dietary trends and the adaptation of existing ones.

The human body is astonishing in its ability to endure and adapt. It processes everything we consume, striving to derive energy from both beneficial and harmful substances. Yet, there's a limit to this resilience. Ignored by many, the body's signals of distress often manifest as various aches and pains. Despite these warnings, we frequently continue our harmful dietary habits.

In my exploration through books, studies, and online communities, certain themes consistently emerged regarding the link between diet and autoimmune diseases: inflammation is often at the root of autoimmune issues and dietary approaches play an important role in exacerbating or alleviating symptoms as well in preventing the advancement of the disease by supporting immune function.

While individual needs vary, here are some diet plans that are commonly recommended for people with autoimmune conditions: Autoimmune Protocol Diet (AIP), Gluten-Free Diet, Paleo Diet, Low-FODMAP Diet, Elimination Diet, Mediterranean Diet. When adopting a new diet, it is important to ensure nutritional needs are met and the approach is tailored to the specific requirements and conditions of each person.

The Autoimmune Protocol (AIP) diet is a more stringent version of the Paleo diet, specifically tailored for individuals with autoimmune disorders. The Paleo diet itself originated from the concepts proposed by Dr. Walter Voegtlin in 1975 and later popularized by Dr. Loren Cordain in 2002. The core philosophy of the Paleo diet involves emulating the dietary habits of our Paleolithic ancestors, focusing on whole foods, and eliminating processed foods, grains, and dairy. The AIP diet goes a step further, aiming to reduce inflammation and heal the gut by removing a broader range of potential inflammatory foods. This diet is particularly relevant for autoimmune conditions since a significant portion of the body's immune cells (around 70 to 80%) are located in the gut. By focusing on gut health, the AIP diet seeks to address the root causes of autoimmune reactions.

Unlike the general Paleo diet, the AIP diet eliminates not only processed foods, grains, and dairy but also nightshades (like tomatoes and eggplants), nuts, seeds, and eggs. These eliminations are based on the premise that these foods might cause inflammation in individuals with a heightened autoimmune response.

Adhering to the AIP diet can be challenging due to its restrictive nature. It often requires a strong motivation, such as the need to manage severe symptoms or control a life-threatening condition, for individuals to commit fully to this dietary change. Despite its challenges, many find the AIP diet beneficial in managing their autoimmune conditions, as it helps in reducing inflammation and promoting gut health. It helps relieve the symptoms for people suffering from several autoimmune diseases like:

- Hashimoto's thyroiditis
- Inflammatory Bowel Disease
- Rheumatoid Arthritis
- Coeliac Disease
- Multiple Sclerosis
- Sjogren's
- Type 1 Diabetes
- Lupus (SLE)

The AIP diet is made up of two phases: the elimination phase and the reintroduction phase. The recommendation is to follow the elimination phase for at least 30 days up to a maximum of 90 days or until symptoms improve.

Upon first encountering the restrictive list of foods permitted during the elimination phase of a diet like AIP, it's natural to feel overwhelmed and concerned. Questions may arise, such as how to sustain a diet without eggs, dairy, legumes, or seeds, what meals can be prepared with such limited ingredients, and how to manage dining out or attending social events and vacations.

Initially, adapting to this change can be quite a shock. However, as time progresses, you learn to create delicious meals within these constraints and discover strategies for selecting AIP-compliant options at restaurants and during travel. The process involves a learning curve, but with experience, navigating these dietary restrictions becomes more manageable and less daunting.

The ingredients believed to be inflammatory, and that AIP diet is eliminating in the first stage are:

- **Grains** - Wheat, barley, oats, rye, corn, rice, quinoa, and other grains.
- **Legumes** - All beans, peas, lentils, quinoa, peanuts.
- **Nightshade vegetables** - Tomatoes, potatoes, eggplants, and peppers.
- **Dairy products** - All milk, cheese, yogurt, and butter (ghee is sometimes allowed).
- **Eggs** - Both the whites and yolks.
- **Nuts and seeds** - All nuts (e.g., almonds, walnuts) and seeds (e.g., flax, chia), as well as seed-derived oils.
- **Processed foods** - Anything processed or with additives, preservatives, artificial colors, or flavors is to be avoided.
- **Refined sugars and oils** - Such as canola oil, sunflower oil, and foods containing refined sugars.
- **Alcohol** - All types of alcoholic beverages are off-limits.
- **Coffee and chocolate.**

- **Certain spices and food additives** - Particularly those derived from seeds and nightshades, such as mustard, paprika, and seed-based culinary oils.

During this phase the focus is to consume whole, unprocessed foods from quality sources of animal protein, healthy fats and organic, nutrient-dense vegetables. Here are the main categories of food allowed during the elimination phase:

- **Vegetables** (excluding nightshades) - Most vegetables are allowed, such as leafy greens, broccoli, cauliflower, cucumbers, zucchini, squash, onions, and garlic.
- **Fruits** - In moderation (typically not more than 2-3 servings per day), including berries, apples, bananas, oranges, and pears.
- **Meats and fish** - Preferably grass-fed, wild, or organic meats like beef, chicken, turkey, pork, and fish such as salmon, mackerel, and sardines.
- **Organ meats** - Liver, heart, and other organ meats are encouraged for their nutrient density.
- **Healthy fats** - Including avocado, olive oil, coconut oil, and avocados.
- Fermented foods - Such as coconut yogurt and fermented vegetables (e.g., sauerkraut and kimchi) that are free from added sugars and not derived from dairy.
- **Herbs and non-seed spices** - Such as turmeric, ginger, and cilantro, which can be used for flavoring.
- **Vinegars** - Like apple cider vinegar and balsamic vinegar, provided they do not contain added sugars.
- **Bone broth** - Highly recommended for its nutrient content and gut-healing properties.
- **Root vegetables and tubers** - Such as sweet potatoes, beets, and carrots.

- **Coconut products** - Including coconut milk, coconut cream, coconut butter, and coconut flakes, as long as they do not contain any additives or sweeteners.
- **Oils** - Coconut oil known for the medium-chain fatty acids and anti-inflammatory properties, olive oil which is high in monounsaturated fats and antioxidants, and avocado oil good for cooking at higher temperatures due to its high smoke point.

At the end of the elimination phase (minimum 30 days or after the symptoms improve) starts the second phase of the AIP diet: reintroduction phase. The goal of this phase is to purposely reintroduce one at a time foods that were eliminated in the first phase identifying thus food sensitivities. Before starting this second phase it is important to ensure that the symptoms have improved significantly and have stabilized during the first phase. This will create a good baseline to compare against each food that is reintroduced. Below is a list with most commonly reintroduced foods:

- Egg yolk
- Legumes sprouted (like lentils and chickpeas)
- Nuts and seeds (in a first phase you can start with nuts and seeds oils and later reintroduce the nuts and seeds as a whole, flours or butters)
- Egg whites
- Other legumes
- Gluten-free grains (like rice and quinoa)
- Potatoes
- Nightshade vegetables (tomatoes, peppers)
- Dairy products (starting with fermented kefir or yogurt)

Each food should be introduced one at a time, over a period of 3-5 days for each. Eat that reintroduced food at least twice each day for the next 3-5 days. During this time, you keep a detailed food diary to track the food reintroduced and monitor for reactions such as:

- Digestive (bloating, gas, abdominal pain/cramps, diarrhea/constipation, changes in bowel habits)
- Skin (rashes, eczema flare-ups, acne, itchy skin, redness or hives)
- Respiratory (sneezing, congestion, asthma exacerbation, nasal back drip)
- Neurological and Emotional (headaches/migraines, fatigue/drowsiness, irritability, anxiety, brain fog, difficulty concentrating)
- Joint and Muscle (pain, swelling, aches, stiffness)
- Systemic Reactions (general feeling unwell, fever, chills, increased inflammation markers).

In the diary it is important to note not only the type of reaction but also the severity and duration. This will help determine if the specific food should be permanently avoided or tried again later. If there is no reaction, the food can be integrated into the diet. If that food triggers a reaction, it should be removed from the diet and possibly tried again later since sometimes sensitivities decrease over time. Allow two, three days for that reaction to clear before going to the next food to be reintroduced. Below is an example of a diary:

Date & time	Food	Digestive (bloating, gas, abdominal pain/cramps, diarrhea, constipation)	Skin (rashes, eczema, acne, itchy skin, redness, hives)	Respiratory (sneezing, congestion, asthma, nasal backdrop)	Neurological (headaches, fatigue, irritability, anxiety, brain fog)	Joints & muscles (pain, swelling, aches, stiffness)	Systemic reactions (fever, chills, feeling unwell)	Other
2/2 08 AM	Egg yolk	None	None	None	Fatigue	Finger joint pain	None	+2 lbs.

Some people might be able to introduce most of the foods that were initially avoided during the elimination phase of the AIP diet. However, for those suffering from an autoimmune disease some foods will have to be avoided forever.

The three most commonly gut-irritating, inflammation-producing foods are gluten, dairy, and sugar. For a complete list of allowed ingredients for the Autoimmune Protocol diet please send me an email at info@aipwellnessjourney.com

According to studies, gluten is producing an inflammatory response even in people with non-celiac sensitivity producing "gastrointestinal distress, fatigue, and pain including inflammation and increased permeability of the intestinal mucosa." [82]. And, as we already know, long term inflammation and the permeability of the intestinal wall (known as leaky gut) leads to a reaction of the innate immune system which in turn leads to the development of different autoimmune diseases. This link between gluten and chronic illnesses has been known for at least a decade now. That is one of the reasons for which more and more people are interested in a healthy diet and more and more products appear on the market bearing the "gluten-free" logo. Some members in certain Facebook groups found that they can digest better and without strong reaction wheat products (pasta and pizza) when they are in Europe as opposed to the same products made with American wheat. It is true that European wheat is different from its American counterpart by its lower gluten content which might explain a lower reaction in people with non-celiac disease. Nonetheless, for individuals already grappling with autoimmune diseases, it may be prudent to completely avoid gluten to mitigate health risks.

Dairy products contain various proteins, including a type called casein, which can sometimes provoke an immune response, potentially leading to inflammation in some individuals. A specific study detailed in the National Library of Medicine [83] involved 45 participants who consumed milk containing different forms of casein—A1 β-casein and A2 β-casein—over separate two-week periods. This study also included a period where participants consumed a blend of both types of casein. The study's results indicated that high intake of milk proteins, especially A1 β-casein, was associated with increased gastrointestinal inflammation. It was observed that this kind of dairy consumption could slow down the digestive process and negatively affect cognitive processing speed and accuracy. This is noteworthy as it suggests a direct link between certain dairy components and digestive and cognitive health.

Furthermore, dairy products are known to be sources of saturated fats. Some research has linked the consumption of saturated fats to heightened inflammation in the body. This aspect is particularly significant as chronic inflammation is a key factor in various health conditions, including cardiovascular diseases and certain autoimmune disorders.

I already talked about the harmful effects of sugar. Just knowing that the cancer cells feed themselves with sugar is incentive enough to stop eating it.

I began the elimination phase of the AIP diet in December 2020, transitioning to the reintroduction phase around March 2021. Initially, I was overwhelmed by the extensive list of foods I had to eliminate, especially since I enjoyed cheese, potatoes, and eggs. I feared I would starve and doubted my ability to adhere to this diet for even a week. However, I underestimated the powerful survival instinct we all possess, and how effectively the fear of chronic illness and pain can motivate us.

Gradually, I adapted to a new way of eating, developing fresh eating habits and finding enjoyment in the challenge of creating new recipes. Cooking had never been my passion, but the challenge of crafting something new each time I entered the kitchen became appealing. By mid-2021, I had successfully reintroduced many of the "forbidden" foods from phase I, yet I continue to avoid gluten, dairy, sugar, soy, nightshades, and largely eggs—though I can incorporate them into baked goods like cake without any adverse reactions. Surprisingly, I don't miss these foods because I've discovered satisfying substitutes and learned to bake bread without the harmful ingredients typically found in store-bought varieties.

Now, let's discuss how to select your daily food in a way that promotes health and helps manage autoimmune symptoms.

4.3 HEALTHY FOOD FOR AUTOIMMUNE DISEASES

Food as medicine or food as poison, it is for us to decide what we want to eat.

What we eat can help us prevent disease, treat or cure us or can be harmful and in the long run can be lethal. Since each of us is unique it is very important to tune into our intuition and observe how our body responds to different foods.

Food is energy, is fuel for our body the same way gasoline is fuel for a car. A balanced diet should include a diverse range of foods to provide our body with the nutrients needed to function optimally. The principles of a balanced diet are:

- Since each food group offers unique benefits, eat different types of foods to ensure you get a wide range of nutrients.

- Moderation is key. While it is important to consume enough of each type of nutrient, too much of any one nutrient can be harmful.

- Ensure that the diet is made of organic fruits and vegetables and quality protein (grass-fed beef, free-range chicken, wild caught seafood).

- Eliminate all pre-processed food, sugar, and read the ingredients to eliminate or minimize the consumption of additives and artificial ingredients.

A balanced diet provides the macronutrients and micronutrients the body needs to function effectively.

The **macronutrients** are needed in larger quantities, and they are carbohydrates, proteins and fats.

The carbohydrates provide the body with energy and they come mainly from grains, fruits, vegetables and some dairy. When carbohydrates we eat are broken down during digestion, glucose is the resulting sugar that gets absorbed into the bloodstream and transported to cells where it is used to produce energy in the form of adenosine triphosphate (ATP). Each carbohydrate provides about 4 calories per gram. Some carbohydrates contain dietary fiber which supports gut health.

Like carbohydrates, the proteins also provide 4 calories per gram, and they are made up of amino acids. They play a critical role in the structure, function and regulation of the body's tissues and organs. Some enzymes and hormones are proteins that catalyze biochemical reactions in the body and, respectively, help regulate various physiological processes. Certain proteins bind and carry atoms and small molecules within cells and the antibodies are proteins that help find infections. There are twenty amino acids in the human body, but our body is able to synthesize only eleven of them. The remaining nine must be obtained from diet and thus their name of essential amino acids. Protein coming from animal food is considered complete because it contains all essential amino acids. Plant-based proteins are lacking one or two of these essential amino acids which is why they are considered incomplete. If you prefer a plant-based diet or an omnivorous diet it is important to experiment with whatever works for your body at the stage, you are right now in your life. It's essential to recognize that we are at the end of the food chain, meaning that we ultimately consume what our food sources, both animal and plant, have ingested or been treated with. For instance, if livestock are fed a diet high in antibiotics and hormones, these substances can potentially enter our bodies when we consume meat. Similarly, the pesticides, herbicides, and fertilizers used on crops can accumulate in plant foods, which we then eat. By choosing foods that are grown and processed responsibly, we can influence the quality of our diets and, consequently, our overall health.

Fats also known as lipids provide 9 calories per gram and they are involved in the synthesis of hormones in the absorption of fat-soluble vitamins such as A, D, E and K and they are important components of cell membranes. Over the years, there has been considerable debate regarding the appropriate quality and quantity of fat in a person's diet. Dietary trends have fluctuated, and many previously popular beliefs, such as the advantages of consuming margarine over butter and choosing low-fat dairy products over full-fat versions, have been debunked.

Good sources of healthy fat are:

- Saturated fatty acids (SFAs): dairy, fatty meat, lard, coconut and cocoa oils
- Monounsaturated fatty acids (MUFAs): avocados, extra-virgin olive oil, nuts, seeds
- Polyunsaturated fatty acids (PUFAs):
- Omega-3: mackerel, salmon, tuna, chia seeds, flaxseeds, walnuts
- Omega-g: nuts, seeds

Trans fatty acids are considered detrimental to health and should be avoided due to their strong links to inflammation, heart disease, and atherosclerosis. Common sources of trans fats include fried foods, frozen pizza, margarine, and processed baked goods. It is advisable to steer clear of food products that list "partially hydrogenated oils" in their ingredients, as these are a major source of trans fats.

The micronutrients are needed in smaller quantities. They are vitamins and minerals that are essential for growth, immune response, hormone regulation and nerve functioning.

There are 13 essential vitamins and can be classified in:

- Fat-soluble: Vitamins A, D, E, and K need to be in the presence of fat to be absorbed and can be stored in the body's tissue.
- Water-soluble: Vitamins B and C dissolve in water and the body eliminates the amounts that are not needed.
- Here are some healthy food sources of vitamins:

- Vitamin A: butter, egg yolks, liver, milk, tuna. Beta-carotene found in squash, pumpkin and carrots can be converted to vitamin A in the body.

- Vitamin D: butter, eggs, liver, fish

- Vitamin E: almonds, avocados, peanuts, spinach, sunflower seeds

- Vitamin K: beet greens, broccoli, cabbage, collards, kale, spinach, turnip greens, Swiss chard

- Vitamin B1 (Thiamin): legumes, nuts, oatmeal, potatoes, pork, seeds

- Vitamin B2 (Riboflavin): almonds, beef, dairy, eggs

- Vitamin B3 (Niacin): chicken, liver, fish, pork, potatoes, turkey

- Vitamin B6: avocado, chicken, chickpeas, liver, navy beans, pistachios, potatoes, salmon, walnuts

- Vitamin B12: beef, eggs, liver, oysters, salmon

- Vitamin C: broccoli, Brussel sprouts, cauliflower, citrus fruits, cranberries, kiwi, potatoes, strawberries, red pepper

Macrominerals and trace minerals are both essential types of minerals that play critical roles in various physiological processes in the body. Macrominerals are needed in larger amounts than trace minerals and they include calcium, phosphorus, magnesium, sodium, potassium, chloride, and sulfur, each with specific roles in our body. Here are some good food sources of macrominerals:

- Calcium: bok choy, cheese, collard greens, kale, milk, sardines, spinach, tofu, yogurt

- Chloride: olives, salt, sea vegetables

- Magnesium: almonds, beans, cashews, flaxseeds, peas, pumpkin seeds, spinach

- Phosphorus: cheese, eggs, lentils, meat, mushrooms, potatoes, sunflower seeds, sardines

- Potassium: bananas, mangoes, milk, oranges, potatoes, squash, tomatoes
- Sodium: celery, eggs, ham, milk, salt, seafood
- Sulfur: beef, eggs, fish, poultry
- Trace minerals are required in smaller amounts but are still vital to health and they include chromium, iron, manganese, copper, iodine, zinc, cobalt, fluoride, and selenium, each serving crucial functions. Here are some healthy food sources of trace minerals:
- Chromium: broccoli, egg yolks, garlic, potatoes, red wine
- Copper: cashews, prunes, sesame seeds
- Fluoride: gelatin, some seafood
- Iodine: cod, eggs, haddock, seaweed
- Iron: beans, lentils, liver, oysters, spinach
- Manganese: almonds, brown rice, beans, pineapple
- Selenium: beef, Brazil nuts, chia seeds, chicken, crab, oysters, pork, salmon, sardines
- Zinc: beef, cashews, chickpeas, oysters, pumpkin seeds, sunflower seeds, crab

So, how do you choose what you eat?

Let's talk about vegetables and fruits.

The most recent US Dietary Guidelines recommend consuming 2-½ cups of vegetables and 2 cups of fruit, based on a 2000-calorie diet.

I am sure you have heard the term "Eat the rainbow". What does it mean? It makes reference to what we put on our plates in terms of color food. Having a colorful plate have a lot of advantages:

- It is full of phytonutrients that maximize our health.
- It makes the food more appetizing through the different colors

- It is an indication that the food you eat is nutrient dense.

The phytonutrients are natural compounds that keep the plant safe from bugs, germs, and other threats. They also give the plant the taste and the aroma. At the human level, due to their anti-inflammatory benefits [108] they affect the cellular structure and function and help us prevent chronic disease and may protect us against different types of cancer [109]. Each color has a different type of phytonutrients that help us at different levels:

- Green vegetables and fruits (spinach, avocados, asparagus, broccoli, kale, cabbage, Brussel sprouts, kiwi, collard greens, lettuce, green herbs like mint, rosemary, sage, thyme and basil) are rich in glucosinolates which are cancer-blocking chemicals.

- Red vegetables and fruits (strawberries, cranberries, raspberries, tomatoes, cherries, apples, beets, watermelon, red grapes, red onions, red peppers) are rich in carotenoid lycopene that may protect against gene-damaging free radicals.

- Orange and yellow vegetables and fruits (carrots, sweet potatoes, yellow peppers, oranges, bananas, pineapple, tangerines, mango, pumpkin, apricots, peaches, cantaloupe, butternut squash, acorn squash) provide beta cryptoxanthin which may prevent heart disease by supporting intracellular communication.

- White and brown vegetables and fruits (onions, cauliflower, garlic, leeks, parsnips, mushrooms, celery root) contain flavonoids like quercetin and kaempferol which have from antioxidant and anti-inflammatory effects to supporting cardiovascular health and potentially reducing cancer risk. Onion and garlic contain allicin which has anti-tumor properties.

- Blue and purple vegetables and fruits (blueberries, blackberries, elderberries, grapes, eggplant, plums, prunes, purple cabbage and cauliflower) are believed to block the formation of blood clots due to their anthocyanins content which is also a powerful antioxidant.

Filling your plate with a variety of colored plants, in other words "eating the rainbow" can be very beneficial for your health.

Another important principle to consider when fighting a chronic disease is to eat organic food. In the case of vegetables and fruits, plants in general, that means to buy plants that are free of synthetic chemicals, in other words they are grown without synthetic pesticides, herbicides or fertilizers; are non-GMO (Genetically Modified Organisms) which means that they are not from genetically modified seeds. An "organic" certification also implies that there are specific standards that must be met during the entire farming, harvesting, and processing of that specific plant.

Cooked or raw?

While in general unprocessed vegetables and fruits help preserve their fiber content and prevent the loss of nutrients that can occur during processing, some nutrients are more available after cooking. It is the case of tomatoes in which the bioavailability of antioxidants like lycopene can increase when cooked.

Cooking vegetables can also be beneficial for people that suffer from certain chronic diseases due to effects on nutrient absorption and digestion.

For example, people with digestive disorders like IBS, Crohn's disease might have issues digesting raw vegetables that can create bloating, gas or abdominal discomfort.

Individuals with hypothyroidism might need to consume some cooked cruciferous vegetables like broccoli, cauliflower, and kale which due to the goitrogens content might inhibit iodine uptake. Cooking them can deactivate the goitrogens making them easier and safer.

In general people with autoimmune conditions and following an AIP diet may benefit from consuming cooked vegetables over raw ones. Cooking can help reduce levels of certain anti-nutrients and compounds like lectins and phytates that might exacerbate symptoms.

Fermenting some vegetables such as cabbage, carrots, cucumber, tomatoes, can reduce the anti-nutrient content. The fermentation process introduces bacteria that can produce enzymes, such as phytase which help break down phytates. It also reduces the levels of oxalates which might be detrimental for people prone to have kidney stones. In addition to the beneficial content in probiotics, the fermentation process makes vegetables easier to digest.

Attention: the fermentation process SHOULD NOT involve vinegar. The natural fermentation process uses naturally occurring lactic acid bacteria present on the vegetable's surface, which convert sugars into lactic acid. Traditional lactic acid fermentation encourages the growth of beneficial bacteria, providing probiotics that support gut health. Vinegar pickling does not involve the growth of beneficial lactic acid bacteria and does not yield these probiotics, limiting thus its health benefits.

Let's move on and talk about legumes.

Legumes are part of phase II of the AIP diet: Reintroduction. They are excluded from the phase I, Elimination, due to their potential harm on the digestive system, leading to potential gut irritation, and gastrointestinal distress such as bloating and gas.

While cruciferous vegetables contain lectins that can be significantly reduced by cooking, the content of lectins in legumes is higher. Lectins are proteins that can bind to cell membranes and potentially interfere with nutrient absorption.

Another anti-nutrient found in legumes, and in smaller proportions in some vegetables like leafy greens and root vegetables, is phytic acid (phytates) which can bind to minerals such as iron, calcium, magnesium and zinc, reducing their bioavailability and reading to nutrient deficiencies.

So how to prepare the legumes?

To reduce their anti-nutrient content and improve digestibility here are some steps that I follow when I prepare legumes:

- Rinsing the legumes under running water helps remove impurities.
- Soaking legumes for several hours (rice, split peas) or overnight (lentils, chickpeas, beans) will help break down oligosaccharides and reduce lectin and phytate content. I

change the water 1-2 times if I soak them for a few hours or every three hours during the day if I soak them overnight. Changing the water helps remove the anti-nutrients.

- Rinsing the legumes after soaking is an important step before starting cooking or sprouting.

- Sprouting lentils, chickpeas, and beans is an excellent way to increase nutrient availability and reduce anti-nutrient content. After soaking and rinsing I drain the legumes, cover them and allow them to germinate in a bowl on the counter. The germination process might take one or up to three, four days, depending on the legume. During this time, I rinse and drain them four, five times each day. When the sprout reaches half an inch, they are ready to be cooked or, for lentils, be used in a flavorful salad.

- Cooking legumes further reduces their anti-nutrient content. Due to my autoimmune disease, I always cook legumes thoroughly.

Let's talk about meat.

As I mentioned previously, regardless if you are or not suffering from a chronic disease, it is important to eat quality meat. Because we are at the end of the food chain, we accumulate both the benefits and potential harms of what the animals we consume have eaten. If the beef, bison, or sheep are grazing on a field treated with pesticides then the meat we will eat will can affect us in different ways:

- The accumulation of pesticide residues in the cow's meat will get ingested by us and thus we will build up those harmful chemicals in our body.

- If we continue ingesting those pesticides over a prolonged period of time, these chemicals can accumulate to higher concentrations in our tissues potentially leading to long-term health issues.

- Pesticide exposure has been linked to health issues such as cancer, hormone disruptions and neurological conditions like Parkinson's disease and cognitive decline.

When choosing the meat to eat we need to consider both the type of meat but also how it is raised and processed.

- **Beef** - Grass-fed animals are primarily raised on grass but may be switched to grains or other feeds towards the end of their lives to increase fat content and alter the flavor of the meat. Grass-fed and grass-finished is considered to be better than only grass-fed. Grass-finished meat tends to be lower in total fat compared to only grass-fed (and grain-finished meat) because it allows the animals to graze in a more natural environment throughout their lives. Organic beef ensures that no synthetic hormones or antibiotics have been used which is better for the animal's health and ours. In summary, organic, grass-fed, grass-finished beef meat is to be considered if you suffer from an autoimmune disease. Unfortunately, this type of meat is very expensive so in case of financial restraints, I would suggest consuming organic, grass-fed beef meat.

- **Poultry** (Chicken and Turkey) - When deciding what poultry meat to buy I suggest organic, pasture-raised. This way you can reduce the exposure to antibiotics and hormones that are used in conventional poultry farming.

- **Fish and seafood** - It is advisable to look for wild-caught seafood. Fish such as salmon, mackerel, sardines are rich in fatty acids which are beneficial for our health. Choosing wild-caught fish we make sure to avoid pigments used to enhance the coloration of the fish, particularly in salmon and antibiotics and medications included in the fish feed to prevent or treat disease.

- **Pork** - As in the Poultry case, you need to look for organic raised pork to avoid meat raised with antibiotics and growth hormones.

- **Game meat** (Venison, Bison) - this type of meat is typically less likely to be raised in confined spaces which results in healthier choice when compared to conventional red meat.

It is generally strongly suggested to eliminate completely or, at least, limit the consumption of processed meat, such as bacon, sausages, deli meats since they are often high in sodium and preservatives which can be linked to increased risk of chronic diseases.

One important concept to follow is eating an animal from "head to tail". This approach refers to consuming every part of the animal, including organs, bones, and skin. In some countries, with traditional diets, people are still eating all parts of an animal using the small and large intestines as well as the stomach to make tasty sausages, UK is known for the kidney pies, heart and liver are used to make stews and pate (spread), head, feet and tail to make cold meals or soups, tongue to make an exceptional olive and tongue meal, brain pane (breaded) is a delicacy in some countries. Unfortunately, all these organs are overlooked in modern diets in western countries. Each part of the animal offers different nutrients, and they are considered nutrient-dense food. Organ meats like liver and kidneys are rich in vitamins and minerals such as iron, vitamin A, and B vitamins. Bones, feet, and ears can be used to make broth which is rich in minerals and collagen and is an important food for gut healing.

Lastly, let's talk about eggs.

When we go to the stores to buy eggs we have to choose between the following types: normal eggs, cage-free, organic, and pasture-raised.

Normal eggs are from chickens raised in conventional cages that restrict chickens' movement. Typically, chickens are subjected to controlled light/no light period of times to increase the fat in the animal.

Cage-free eggs indicate that the chickens are not raised in confined conditions, but they still don't have access to the outdoors. They are able to walk and spread their wings, but they are still in a crowded environment, and they don't see the sun.

Organic eggs come from chickens that are fed an organic diet, free from pesticides, synthetic fertilizers, and GMOs and typically, are raised without antibiotics or growth hormones.

Pasture-raised eggs come from chickens that are allowed to roam freely outdoors on a pasture where they can forage for their natural diet which includes seeds, plants, insects, and worms. Typically pasture-raised eggs have higher levels of omega-3 fatty acids and vitamins, and the color of the yolk is more intense.

My suggestion when choosing eggs is to go for organic, pasture-raised eggs which are more beneficial for our health.

4.4 FOOD LABELS AND INGREDIENTS

Know what you eat; read the label before you buy.

Knowing how to read the food labels is essential to understanding what it is in the food and beverages we buy and consume, and it helps us make healthy decisions. Food labels can be complex, so it's valuable to discuss and clarify some key aspects.

A food label provides essential information, such as nutrition facts, which are straightforward, the "best if used by" date which indicates optimal freshness. It also includes claims like organic, low-fat, and low-calorie, or specifies if the product is grass-fed, offering guidance on its quality and suitability for various dietary preferences.

Produce often has a PLU code: a four-digit code beginning with 3 or 4 indicates conventional farming methods, while a five-digit code starting with 9 denotes organic produce.

The ingredient list is also essential; it shows everything the product contains, listed in descending order by weight. The first listed ingredient is the most predominant in the product, and the last listed ingredient is the least. In other words, the ingredient that weighs the most, therefore has the most percentage content is listed first and the ingredient that weighs least, therefore has the least percentage content is listed last. The first three ingredients make up the majority of the content of the product. As a rule of thumb, the foods that have the shortest list of ingredients are considered better choices due to fewer additives and preservatives.

INGREDIENTS:
Organic Coconut Meat, Organic Coconut Water, Organic Virgin Coconut Oil.
Contains Tree Nuts (Coconut)

INGRÉDIENTS:
Noix de coco biologique. Eau de noix de coco biologique. Huile vierge de noix de coco biologique.
Contient des noix de coco.

In the attached label the whole list of ingredients is very healthy: coconut meat, coconut water and coconut oil, all organic. This is a safe product to buy.

Ingredients: Sugars* (invert cane syrup*), Gluten free flour blend* (oat flour*, tapioca starch*, ground chia seeds*), Palm fruit oil*†, Vanilla chips* (cocoa butter*, cane sugar*, tapioca starch*, rice syrup solids*, rice maltodextrin*, vanilla extract*), Sunflower oil*, Vegetable glycerin*, Natural flavours*, Baking powder, Beet powder*, Cocoa powder*, Vegetable extracts (spinach, broccoli, carrots, tomatoes, beets, shiitake mushrooms), Sea salt.
*Organic. †Sustainable.

Ingrédients: Sucres* (sirop de canne inverti*), Mélange de farine sans gluten* (farine d'avoine*, fécule de tapioca*, graines de chia moulues*), Huile de palme*†, Pépites
flc
sh

INGREDIENTS: Enriched wheat flour (wheat, barley, niacin, reduced iron, thiamine mononitrate, riboflavin, folic acid), sugar, chocolate chunks (sugar, chocolate liquor, cocoa butter, soy lecithin, vanilla, salt), brown sugar, vegetable oil blend (palm fruit, soybean and olive oils, water, salt, non-fat milk, mono and diglycerides, soy lecithin, potassium sorbate as a preservative, natural and artificial flavor, vitamin A palmitate, beta carotene color), butter, eggs, invert sugar, soy flour, salt, baking soda, natural vanilla flavor..

The first ingredient in the label is sugar. Even though it is specified "organic" the cane sugar syrup is not AIP compliant. The next two ingredients are gluten free flour blend and palm fruit oil. What this label is telling us is that we mainly eat a lot of sugar mixed with rs and vegetable extracts ng this product.

This product is very healthy, but it is not AIP compliant due to the chia seed content. If you are in the Introduction phase and you already introduced chia seeds without any side effect, then this is a very good product to consume.

This is another example of a product that is not healthy. The first three ingredients are enriched wheat flour, sugar, and chocolate chunks. It does not bring us any healthy nutritive value. In addition, the soybean oils, mono and diglycerides, soy lecithin, potassium sorbate, natural and artificial flavor, and natural vanilla flavor, amongst others are alarm signals for someone who wants to follow a healthy diet.

Ingredients: Cassava blend (cassava flour, cassava starch), Avocado oil, Coconut flour, Chia seed, Sea salt.

Ingrédients : Mélange de manioc (farine de manioc, amidon de manioc), Huile d'avocat, Farine de noix de coco, Graines de chia, Sel de mer.

It's important to be vigilant about ingredients listed on food labels, especially various forms of sugars and sweeteners, such as sugar, corn sweetener, corn syrup, dextrose, fructose, and cornstarch. These ingredients are often added to processed foods and can significantly increase the sugar content without adding nutritional value. Many consumers are unaware of the various names that sugar can be listed under on food labels. Besides the ones mentioned, sugar can also appear as maltose, sucrose, high-fructose corn syrup, barley malt, and more.

In addition to sugars there are several other ingredients commonly found on product labels that are best consumed in moderation or avoided due to potential health risks:

Trans Fats, often listed as "partially hydrogenated oils", are associated with an increased risk of heart disease, stroke, and type 2 diabetes. They can raise bad cholesterol levels (LDL) and lower good cholesterol levels (HDL).

Artificial Sweeteners such as aspartame, sucralose, saccharin, and acesulfame potassium are linked to weight gain and glucose intolerance, and they may negatively affect gut microbiota.

Sodium Nitrate/Nitrite, commonly used in cured meats like bacon, sausages, and deli meats, helps preserve food and enhance color. However, they can convert into nitrosamines in the body, potentially leading to an increased risk of cancer.

Artificial Colors ingredients such as Red 40, Yellow 5, and Blue 1 are used to enhance the appearance of foods. Concerns about artificial colors include links to behavioral issues in children and possible carcinogenic effects.

Monosodium Glutamate (MSG) is used as a flavor enhancer. MSG can cause headaches and other symptoms in some individuals, commonly referred to as "MSG symptom complex."

High Fructose Corn Syrup (HFCS), found in many processed foods and beverages, is linked to obesity, diabetes, fatty liver disease, and inflammation.

Artificial Flavors, while they mimic natural flavors, are chemical compounds created in a lab. While generally recognized as safe, the long-term health impacts of some synthetic flavoring agents remain uncertain.

Natural Flavors, while the original source of natural flavors must be plant or animal material, can be highly processed and contain many chemical additives. As long as the food manufacturers list "flavors", natural or artificial on ingredients lists, they are not required to reveal the original sources or chemical mixtures of these flavors.

Preservatives such as BHA, BHT, and propyl gallate are used to extend the shelf life of foods but may pose health risks, including potential effects on hormone function and increased cancer risk.

Seed oils such as sunflower oil, safflower oil, sesame oil, canola oil, corn oil, soybean oil, are high in omega-6 polyunsaturated fatty acids which might produce an imbalance between omega-6 and omega-3 fatty acids in the body, leading to inflammation. We already know that inflammation is a risk factor for chronic diseases. In addition, most seed oils undergo extensive processing using high heat, deodorizers and chemical solvents which can create free radicals known to be harmful to health. The high heat used in processing these oils can cause some of the fatty acids in these oils to become trans fats, associated with an increased risk of cardiovascular diseases.

Starting the AIP elimination diet can be daunting for many people and very difficult to follow if it is started brusquely. If this is your case, feel free to start small. Crowd out highly processed foods, added sugars, seed oils and artificial sweeteners. As you crowd out these foods, consider adding in sources of prebiotics such as garlic and onion, and gut-friendly, probiotic-rich fermented foods such as kimchi, sauerkraut, brine pickles. It is also helpful to include food high in inflammation-fighting omega-3 fatty acids such as fatty fish which promote the growth of bacteria, as well as polyphenols found in vegetables and fruits which may increase the healthy flora in your gut microbiome. "Eat the rainbow" when you fill your plate with whole, nutrient-dense food. Eat with intention: home-cooked, seasonal, organic foods: leafy greens, fatty fish, good quality meat and organs, berries and vegetables.

My approach was to start the elimination diet "cold turkey". It helped me adapt faster to the new reality of my new diet. I also adopted an 18-6 intermittent fasting, eating only two nutrient-dense foods, incorporating healthy proteins from organic meat and organs. I completely eliminated snacking in-between the meals. This allowed the Migrating Motor Complex (MMC) to function appropriately. The MMC are cleaning waves that sweep through the intestines. The main role of MMC is to clear undigested food and bacteria from the stomach and small intestines into the large intestine, preventing bacterial overgrowth into the small intestine and maintaining a healthy balance of gut microbiota. These waves work only in a fasted state, typically lasting about 90 to 120 minutes. If we constantly eat or snack, the MMC cannot do its job and bacteria can build up, fermentation can happen and inflammation in the intestines might develop.

One important factor in being successful in your new reality is your mindset: approach diet as a lifestyle and not as a diet regimen for a short-term purpose like losing weight.

Living and thriving with an autoimmune disease is possible. It only requires you to be mindful about your lifestyle, including the skincare products you use, stress management and the diet you follow. I cannot stress enough the importance of being well informed and being an advocate for yourself when needed.

REFERENCES

1. https://autoimmune.org/
2. https://www.health.harvard.edu/diseases-and-conditions/autoimmunity-indicators-on-the-rise-among-americans
3. https://www.autoimmuneinstitute.org/resources/autoimmune-disease-list/
4. https://pubmed.ncbi.nlm.nih.gov/28186008/
5. Imhann F, Bonder MJ, Vich Vila A, Fu J, Mujagic Z, Vork L, Tigchealaar EF, Jankipersadsing SA, Cenit MC, Harmsen HJ, Dijkstra G, Franke L, Zavier RJ, Jonkers D, Wijmenga C, WEersma RK, Zhernakova A. Proton pump inhibitors affect the gut microbiome. Gut. 2016 May;65(5):740-8. Doi: 10.1136/gutjnl-2015-310376. Epub 2015 Dec 9. PMID : 26657899; PMC4853569.
6. Daher R, Yazbeck T, Jaoude JB, Abboud B. Consequences of dysthyroidism on the digestive tract and viscera. World Journal of Gastroenterology. 2009;15(23):2834-2838. doi:10.3748/wjg.15.2834
7. He W, An X, Li L, Shao X, Li Q, Yao Q, Zhang JA. Relationship between Hypothyroidism and Non-Alcoholic Fatty Liver Disease: A Systematic Review and Meta-analysis. Front Endocrinol (Lausanne). 2017 Nov 29;8:335. doi: 10.3389/fendo.2017.00335. PMID: 29238323; PMCID: PMC5712538
8. Iglesias P, Bajo MA, Selgas R, Díez JJ. Thyroid dysfunction and kidney disease: An update. Rev Endocr Metab Disord. 2017 Mar;18(1):131-144. doi: 10.1007/s11154-016-9395-7. PMID: 27864708.
9. Bernal J. Thyroid Hormones in Brain Development and Function. [Updated 2022 Jan 14]. In: Feingold KR, Anawalt B, Blackman MR, et al., editors. Endotext [Internet]. South Dartmouth (MA): MDText.com, Inc.; 2000-. Available from: https://www.ncbi.nlm.nih.gov/books/NBK285549/
10. Gupta N, Arora M, Sharma R, Arora KS. Peripheral and

Central Nervous System Involvement in Recently Diagnosed Cases of Hypothyroidism: An Electrophysiological Study. Ann Med Health Sci Res. 2016 Sep-Oct;6(5):261-266. doi: 10.4103/amhsr.amhsr_39_16. PMID: 28503341; PMCID: PMC5414436.
11. https://www.nei.nih.gov/learn-about-eye-health/eye-conditions-and-diseases/graves-eye-disease
12. Khan R, Sikanderkhel S, Gui J, Adeniyi AR, O'Dell K, Erickson M, Malpartida J, Mufti Z, Khan T, Mufti H, Al-Adwan SA, Alvarez D, Davis J, Pendley J, Patel D. Thyroid and Cardiovascular Disease: A Focused Review on the Impact of Hyperthyroidism in Heart Failure. Cardiol Res. 2020 Apr;11(2):68-75. doi: 10.14740/cr1034. Epub 2020 Mar 10. PMID: 32256913; PMCID: PMC7092768.
13. G. E. Krassas, K. Poppe, D. Glinoer, Thyroid Function and Human Reproductive Health, Endocrine Reviews, Volume 31, Issue 5, 1 October 2010, Pages 702–755, https://doi.org/10.1210/er.2009-0041
14. Cakir M, Samanci N, Balci N, Balci MK. Musculoskeletal manifestations in patients with thyroid disease. Clin Endocrinol (Oxf). 2003 Aug;59(2):162-7. doi: 10.1046/j.1365-2265.2003.01786.x. PMID: 12864792.
15. Yaylali O, Kirac S, Yilmaz M, Akin F, Yuksel D, Demirkan N, Akdag B. Does hypothyroidism affect gastrointestinal motility? Gastroenterol Res Pract. 2009;2009:529802. doi: 10.1155/2009/529802. Epub 2010 Mar 7. PMID: 20224642; PMCID: PMC2833301.
16. Lauritano AC, Bilotta AL, Gabrielli M, Scarpellini E, Lupascu A, Laginestra A, et al. Association between hypothyroidism and small intestinal bacterial overgrowth. J Clin Endocrinol Metab. 2007;92(11):4180-4184.
17. Chen CH, Lin CL, Kao CH. Association between Hashimoto's thyroiditis and cholelithiasis: a retrospective cohort study in Taiwan. BMJ Open. 2018 Sep 5;8(9):e020798. doi: 10.1136/bmjopen-2017-020798. PMID: 30185568; PMCID: PMC6129049.
18. Knezevic J, Starchl C, Tmava Berisha A, Amrein K. Thyroid-Gut-Axis: How Does the Microbiota Influence Thyroid Function? Nutrients. 2020 Jun 12;12(6):1769. doi:

10.3390/nu12061769. PMID: 32545596; PMCID: PMC7353203.
19. Saffouri, G.B., Shields-Cutler, R.R., Chen, J. et al. Small intestinal microbial dysbiosis underlies symptoms associated with functional gastrointestinal disorders. Nat Commun 10, 2012 (2019). https://doi.org/10.1038/s41467-019-09964-7
20. 83 - Fasano A. Leaky gut and autoimmune diseases. Clin Rev Allergy Immunol. 2012 Feb;42(1):71-8. doi: 10.1007/s12016-011-8291-x. PMID: 22109896.
21. 84- Mu Q, Kirby J, Reilly CM, Luo XM. Leaky Gut As a Danger Signal for Autoimmune Diseases. Front Immunol. 2017 May 23;8:598. doi: 10.3389/fimmu.2017.00598. PMID: 28588585; PMCID: PMC5440529.
22. 85 -Song H, Zhu J, Lu D. Long-term proton pump inhibitor (PPI) use and the development of gastric pre-malignant lesions. Cochrane Database of Systematic Reviews 2014, Issue 12. Art. No.: CD010623. DOI: 10.1002/14651858.CD010623.pub2. Accessed 26 November 2023.
23. 86 -Shah SC, Gawron AJ, Li D. Surveillance of Gastric Intestinal Metaplasia. Am J Gastroenterol. 2020 May;115(5):641-644. doi: 10.14309/ajg.0000000000000540. PMID: 32058339; PMCID: PMC7364865.
24. Lash JG, Genta RM. Adherence to the Sydney System guidelines increases the detection of Helicobacter gastritis and intestinal metaplasia in 400738 sets of gastric biopsies. Aliment Pharmacol Ther. 2013 Aug;38(4):424-31. doi: 10.1111/apt.12383. Epub 2013 Jun 24. PMID: 23796212.
25. 88
https://www.sciencedirect.com/science/article/abs/pii/S0210570523003916
26. Barrett's Esophagus | NIDDK (nih.gov)
27. https://www.mayoclinic.org/diseases-conditions/barretts-esophagus/symptoms-causes/syc-20352841
28. Ireland CJ, Thompson SK, Laws TA, Esterman A. Risk factors for Barrett's esophagus: a scoping review. Cancer Causes Control. 2016 Mar;27(3):301-23. doi: 10.1007/s10552-015-0710-5. Epub 2016 Feb 5. PMID: 26847374.

29. Stress and Thyroid Autoimmunity. Tetsuya Mizokami, Audrey Wu Li, Samer El-Kaissi, and Jack R. Wall https://www.liebertpub.com/doi/abs/10.1089/thy.2004.14.1047
30. https://www.ncbi.nlm.nih.gov/pmc/articles/PMC5579396/
31. Ayazi S, Leers JM, Oezcelik A, Abate E, Peyre CG, Hagen JA, DeMeester SR, Banki F, Lipham JC, DeMeester TR, Crookes PF. Measurement of gastric pH in ambulatory esophageal pH monitoring. Surg Endosc. 2009 Sep;23(9):1968-73. doi: 10.1007/s00464-008-0218-0. Epub 2008 Dec 6. PMID: 19067071.
32. https://www.ncbi.nlm.nih.gov/books/NBK547892/#ProtonPumpInhibitors.OVERVIEW
33. Imhann F, Bonder MJ, Vich Vila A, Fu J, Mujagic Z, Vork L, Tigchelaar EF, Jankipersadsing SA, Cenit MC, Harmsen HJ, Dijkstra G, Franke L, Xavier RJ, Jonkers D, Wijmenga C, Weersma RK, Zhernakova A. Proton pump inhibitors affect the gut microbiome. Gut. 2016 May;65(5):740-8. doi: 10.1136/gutjnl-2015-310376. Epub 2015 Dec 9. PMID: 26657899; PMCID: PMC4853569.
34. IBS Facts and Statistics - About IBS
35. Singh H, Meyer AN, Thomas EJ. The frequency of diagnostic errors in outpatient care: estimations from three large observational studies involving US adult populations. BMJ Qual Saf. 2014 Sep;23(9):727-31. doi: 10.1136/bmjqs-2013-002627. Epub 2014 Apr 17. PMID: 24742777; PMCID: PMC4145460.
36. The great cholesterol myth, by Jonny Bowen, Ph.D, C.N.S and Stephen Sinatra M.D., F.A.C.C.
37. https://www.ncbi.nlm.nih.gov/books/NB
38. K547929/32. https://medlineplus.gov/ency/patientinstructions/000381.htm
39. Why Stomach Acid is Good for you: Natural Relief from Heartburn, Indigestion, Reflux and GERD, by Jonathan Wrigth & Lane Lenard
40. https://www.healthline.com/nutrition/licorice-root#uses
41. pH Scale | U.S. Geological Survey (usgs.gov)

42. https://www.clinicaleducation.org/resources/reviews/the-role-of-hcl-in-gastric-function-and-health/#_ftn1
43. Hsu M, Safadi AO, Lui F. Physiology, Stomach. [Updated 2021 Jul 22]. In: StatPearls [Internet]. Treasure Island (FL): StatPearls Publishing; 2022 Jan-. Available from: https://www.ncbi.nlm.nih.gov/books/NBK535425/
44. https://www.britannica.com/science/human-digestive-system
45. Hirschowitz BI. Pepsinogen. Postgrad Med J. 1984;60(709):743-750. doi:10.1136/pgmj.60.709.743
46. Piper DW, Fenton BH. pH stability and activity curves of pepsin with special reference to their clinical importance. Gut. 1965;6(5):506-508. doi:10.1136/gut.6.5.506
47. The Digestive Process: How Is Food Digested in the Stomach? | University Hospitals (uhhospitals.org)
48. US FDA/CFSAN - Approximate pH of Foods and Food Products (webpal.org)
49. https://en.wikipedia.org/wiki/Secretin
50. DiGregorio N, Sharma S. Physiology, Secretin. [Updated 2021 May 9]. In: StatPearls [Internet]. Treasure Island (FL): StatPearls Publishing; 2022 Jan-. Available from: https://www.ncbi.nlm.nih.gov/books/NBK537116/
51. Guilliams, Thomas G, and Lindsey E Drake. "Meal-Time Supplementation with Betaine HCl for Functional Hypochlorhydria: What is the Evidence?." Integrative medicine (Encinitas, Calif.) vol. 19,1 (2020): 32-36.
52. Feldman M, Barnett C. Fasting gastric pH and its relationship to true hypochlorhydria in humans. Dig Dis Sci. 1991 Jul;36(7):866-9. doi: 10.1007/BF01297133. PMID: 2070698.
53. Force RW, Nahata MC. Effect of histamine H2-receptor antagonists on vitamin B12 absorption. Ann Pharmacother. 1992 Oct;26(10):1283-6. doi: 10.1177/106002809202601018. PMID: 1358279.
54. http://healthyeating.sfgate.com/deficiency-amino-acids-can-cause-conditions-2972.html
55. Li P, Yin YL, Li D, Kim SW, Wu G. Amino acids and immune function. Br J Nutr. 2007 Aug;98(2):237-52. doi: 10.1017/S000711450769936X. Epub 2007 Apr 3. PMID: 17403271.

56. Riccio P, Rossano R. Undigested Food and Gut Microbiota May Cooperate in the Pathogenesis of Neuroinflammatory Diseases: A Matter of Barriers and a Proposal on the Origin of Organ Specificity. Nutrients. 2019;11(11):2714. Published 2019 Nov 9. doi:10.3390/nu11112714
57. https://www.drhagmeyer.com/overlooked-symptoms-of-low-stomach-acid-whos-at-risk/
58. Tennant, Sharon M et al. "Influence of gastric acid on susceptibility to infection with ingested bacterial pathogens." Infection and immunity vol. 76,2 (2008): 639-45. doi:10.1128/IAI.01138-07
59. https://www.nih.gov/news-events/nih-research-matters/blocking-stomach-acid-may-promote-chronic-liver-disease
60. https://www.realizehealth.com.au/2017/07/11/it-all-starts-with-stomach-acid/
61. https://emedicine.medscape.com/article/170066-overview
62. McColl KE. Effect of proton pump inhibitors on vitamins and iron. Am J Gastroenterol. 2009 Mar;104 Suppl 2:S5-9. doi: 10.1038/ajg.2009.45. PMID: 19262546.
63. Fatima R, Aziz M. Achlorhydria. [Updated 2022 May 1]. In: StatPearls [Internet]. Treasure Island (FL): StatPearls Publishing; 2022 Jan-. Available from: https://www.ncbi.nlm.nih.gov/books/NBK507793/
64. Jonathan V. Wright, M.D., Lane Lenard, Ph.D., Why stomach acid is good for you. Natural Relief from Heartburn, Indigestion, Reflux, and GERD.
65. https://www.webmd.com/digestive-disorders/what-is-hypochlorhydria
66. https://www.cghjournal.org/article/S1542-3565(20)30275-5/fulltext?rss=yes#
67. Obrenovich MEM. Leaky Gut, Leaky Brain? Microorganisms. 2018 Oct 18;6(4):107. doi: 10.3390/microorganisms6040107. PMID: 30340384; PMCID: PMC6313445.
68. Lin SH, Chang YS, Lin TM, et al. Proton Pump Inhibitors Increase the Risk of Autoimmune Diseases: A Nationwide Cohort Study. Front Immunol. 2021;12:736036. Published 2021 Sep 30. doi:10.3389/fimmu.2021.736036

69. Protein Deficiency: 7 Signs You're Not Getting Enough Protein (webmd.com)
70. Ahmed A, Clarke JO. Proton Pump Inhibitors (PPI) [Updated 2022 May 8]. In: StatPearls [Internet]. Treasure Island (FL): StatPearls Publishing; 2022 Jan-. Available from: https://www.ncbi.nlm.nih.gov/books/NBK557385/
71. https://www.ncbi.nlm.nih.gov/pmc/articles/PMC9577826/
72. Sipponen P, Härkönen M. Hypochlorhydric stomach: a risk condition for calcium malabsorption and osteoporosis? Scand J Gastroenterol. 2010;45(2):133-8. doi: 10.3109/00365520903434117. PMID: 19958055
73. Sharma VR, Brannon MA, Carloss EA. Effect of omeprazole on oral iron replacement in patients with iron deficiency anemia. South Med J. 2004 Sep;97(9):887-9. doi: 10.1097/01.SMJ.0000110405.63179.69. PMID: 15455980.
74. Ito, T., Jensen, R.T. Association of Long-Term Proton Pump Inhibitor Therapy with Bone Fractures and Effects on Absorption of Calcium, Vitamin B12, Iron, and Magnesium. Curr Gastroenterol Rep 12, 448–457 (2010). https://doi.org/10.1007/s11894-010-0141-0
75. Sturniolo GC, Montino MC, Rossetto L, Martin A, D'Inca R, D'Odorico A, Naccarato R. Inhibition of gastric acid secretion reduces zinc absorption in man. J Am Coll Nutr. 1991 Aug;10(4):372-5. doi: 10.1080/07315724.1991.10718165. PMID: 1894892.
76. Common Acid Reflux Medications Promote Chronic Liver Disease (ucsd.edu)
77. Bloating and poor digestion? Three causes of low pancreatic enzymes | Dr. K. News (drknews.com)
78. Diagnose EPI in Your Patients | Symptom Info For HCPs (identifyepi.com)
79. Low Stomach Acid: What Causes it + How to know if you have it - Back To The Book Nutrition
80. Pancreatic Enzyme Deficiency – Causes, Symptoms, Pancreas Tests | Healthhype.com
81. Pyo JH, Kim TJ, Lee H, Choi SC, Cho SJ, Choi YH, Min YW, Min BH, Lee JH, Kang M, Lee YC, Kim JJ. Proton pump inhibitors use and the risk of fatty liver disease: A nationwide

cohort study. J Gastroenterol Hepatol. 2021 May;36(5):1235-1243. doi: 10.1111/jgh.15236. Epub 2020 Oct 22. PMID: 32886822.
82. Philip A, White ND. Gluten, Inflammation, and Neurodegeneration. Am J Lifestyle Med. 2022 Jan 11;16(1):32-35. doi: 10.1177/15598276211049345. PMID: 35185424; PMCID: PMC8848113.
83. Jianqin S, Leiming X, Lu X, Yelland GW, Ni J, Clarke AJ. Effects of milk containing only A2 beta casein versus milk containing both A1 and A2 beta casein proteins on gastrointestinal physiology, symptoms of discomfort, and cognitive behavior of people with self-reported intolerance to traditional cows' milk. Nutr J. 2016 Apr 2;15:35. doi: 10.1186/s12937-016-0147-z. Erratum in: Nutr J. 2016;15(1):45. PMID: 27039383; PMCID: PMC4818854.
84. 5https://ijpsr.com/bft-article/artificial-preservatives-and-their-harmful-effects-looking-toward-nature-for-safer-alternatives/
85. Evidence of sugar addiction: Behavioral and neurochemical effects of intermittent, excessive sugar intake. https://www.ncbi.nlm.nih.gov/pmc/articles/PMC2235907/
86. https://www.nih.gov/news-events/nih-research-matters/high-sugar-intake-worsens-autoimmune-disease-mice
87. https://www.health.harvard.edu/blog/artificial-sweeteners-sugar-free-but-at-what-cost-201207165030
88. Medical news today https://www.medicalnewstoday.com/articles/146677#effects
89. Morris MJ, Na ES, Johnson AK. Salt craving:the psychobiology of pathogenic sodium intake. Physiol Behav. 2008 Aug 6;94(5):709-21. doi: 10.1016/j.physbeh.2008.04.008. Epub 2008 Apr 13. PMID: 18514747; PMCID: PMC2491403
90. https://www.health.harvard.edu/staying-healthy/why-stress-causes-people-to-overeat
91. http://www.vivo.colostate.edu/hbooks/pathphys/digestion/basics/transit.html

92. https://www.nia.nih.gov/news/research-intermittent-fasting-shows-health-benefits
93. https://www.ncbi.nlm.nih.gov/pmc/articles/PMC4056176/#B3
94. Hippocrates. Hippocrates: With an English Translation by W.H.S. Jones
95. https://www.sciencedirect.com/science/article/abs/pii/S1568997217302835?via%3Dihub
96. https://www.ncbi.nlm.nih.gov/pmc/articles/PMC7700832/
97. https://academic.oup.com/sleep/article/38/4/581/2416911
98. https://www.cdc.gov/chronicdisease/resources/publications/factsheets/nutrition.htm
99. https://www.hsph.harvard.edu/news/hsph-in-the-news/doctors-nutrition-education/
100. https://blogs.bmj.com/bmj/2016/06/16/peter-c-gotzsche-prescription-drugs-are-the-third-leading-cause-of-death/
101. https://ourworldindata.org/data-review-air-pollution-deaths
102. https://www.statista.com/statistics/1137375/air-pollution-deaths-united-states/
103. https://www.ncbi.nlm.nih.gov/pmc/articles/PMC6141690/
104. https://pubmed.ncbi.nlm.nih.gov/28436478/
105. https://www.nrdc.org/issues/toxic-chemicals
106. https://www.safecosmetics.org
107. Pollard KM, Cauvi DM, Toomey CB, Hultman P, Kono DH. Mercury-induced inflammation and autoimmunity. Biochim Biophys Acta Gen Subj. 2019 Dec;1863(12):129299. doi: 10.1016/j.bbagen.2019.02.001. Epub 2019 Feb 10. PMID: 30742953; PMCID: PMC6689266.
https://www.ncbi.nlm.nih.gov/pmc/articles/PMC6689266/
108. Shankar, S., Kumar, D., & Srivastava, R. K. (2013). Epigenetic modifications by dietary phytochemicals: Implications for personalized nutrition. Pharmacol Ther

138(1), 1–17. doi.org/10.1016/j.pharmthera.2012.11.002
109. Zhang, Y. J., Gan, R. Y., Li, S., Zhou, Y., Li, A. N., Xu, D. P., & Li, H. B. (2015). Antioxidant phytochemicals for the prevention and treatment of chronic diseases. Molecules 20(12), 21138–21156. doi.org/10.3390/molecules201219753
110. Mar-Solís LM, Soto-Domínguez A, Rodríguez-Tovar LE, Rodríguez-Rocha H, García-García A, Aguirre-Arzola VE, Zamora-Ávila DE, Garza-Arredondo AJ, Castillo-Velázquez U. Analysis of the Anti-Inflammatory Capacity of Bone Broth in a Murine Model of Ulcerative Colitis. Medicina (Kaunas). 2021 Oct 20;57(11):1138. doi: 10.3390/medicina57111138. PMID: 34833355; PMCID: PMC8618064.
111. K.A. Steinmetz et al., American Journal of Epidemiology: "Vegetables, fruit, and colon cancer in the Iowa Women's Health Study."
112. H. Kim et al., International Journal of Cancer: "Garlic intake and gastric cancer risk: Results from two large prospective US cohort studies."
113. A.A. Myneni et al., Cancer Epidemiology, Biomarkers & Prevention: "Raw Garlic Consumption and Lung Cancer in a Chinese Population."
114. American Institute for Cancer Research: "AICR's Foods That Fight Cancer."

AUTHOR BIO

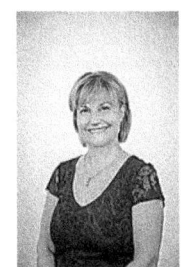 Ionelia Silvia Prajescu is a mechanical engineer with a rich international background, having lived and worked in Romania, Canada, Mexico, and the United States over the span of her accomplished career. Her journey into the realm of health began following a series of stressful relocations and workplace changes, which led to severe stomach pain and eventually to a diagnosis of autoimmune diseases. These health challenges were compounded by diagnostic errors and prolonged use of acid-suppressing medications, resulting in gut dysbiosis, and acquired autoimmune conditions.

Frustrated by the conventional medical field's dismissal of her symptoms as psychosomatic, Silvia took control of her health. She embarked on a profound journey to understand the root causes of her ailments, transforming her life through diet and lifestyle modifications. Today, she manages her autoimmune conditions effectively without reliance on harsh medications.

In 2020, recognizing the sense of helplessness that often accompanies such diagnoses, Silvia was motivated to empower others. She became a **certified Integrative Nutrition Health Coach**, applying her engineering mindset to unravel the complexities of the human body and advocate for foundational health strategies that address inflammation—the core of many autoimmune diseases.

Her book aims to support those who feel overlooked by traditional healthcare, guiding them towards reclaiming their health through informed, sustainable changes. Silvia champions the use of lifestyle adjustments and diet as primary tools for combating autoimmune diseases, advocating for thoughtful, personalized approaches to health before turning to more invasive treatments.

www.ingramcontent.com/pod-product-compliance
Lightning Source LLC
Chambersburg PA
CBHW052028030426
42337CB00027B/4911